Christian Revival Diet™

A personal Journey

Deconstruct to Reconstruct:
Healthy Habits and
seeking revival in Christ

By D. Duane Engler

1 Corinthians 6:19-20

"Do you not know that your bodies are temples of the Holy Spirit, who is in you, whom you have received from God? You are not your own; you were bought with a price. Therefore honor God with your bodies."

Unless noted all Bible verses are from the following sources.

The Holy Bible, New International Version®, NIV® Copyright 1973,
1978, 1984, 2011 by Biblica, Inc. ™ Used by permission. All rights
reserved worldwide.

This book is not a health recommendation or any form of
prescription, nor should be taken as specific medical advice. Please
consult your Physician and/or health care professional about your
specific needs before trying any of the listed items in the book. Make
sure that a professional in the subject matter has deemed you fit
enough to try any of these things.

This book is for general reflection purposes and open for
interpretation. Your specific health needs, history, and functionality
may dictate halting, avoiding or stopping any of the items addressed
through this book.

ISBN-13: 978-1494499389
ISBN-10: 149449938X

A GIFT TO:

FROM:

DEDICATION

This book is dedicated to my Mother and Father who raised me to love Jesus and to continually strive and seek Him in all I do.

I lift this book up in prayer to Jesus.

Mom and Dad,
Your love for me reflects in everything that I do. There are so fond memories we share, as I teach my children, I appreciate those memories more and more everyday.

Your role modeling of awesome Christ centered nutritional tips and patient persistence in implementing positive change is something for which I can't thank you enough.

May this book bless my children and wife as they continue to love and support me in my striving despite my many faults, challenges, and sins.

Twenty Percent of all profits from this book will be donated to global missions that promote spreading the whole gospel, grace and repentance, of Jesus Christ, with a hope for sparking great revival.

To God be the glory!

With Love,
D. Duane Engler

For at the end of all the travels, you may return to where you started and finally know the value of where you started and why such a mission knocked on your door to journey in the first place. Whether it's your journey to the local grocery store or around the world.

"Finally, brothers and sisters, whatever is true, whatever is noble, whatever is right, whatever is pure, whatever is lovely, whatever is admirable—if anything is excellent or praiseworthy—think about such things.

Whatever you have learned or received or heard from me, or seen in me—put it into practice. And the God of peace will be with you."

Philippians 4:8-9

CONTENTS

When at first you don't succeed…..

Pray

Think

Do (read your Bible)

Consider

Wait

Pray again

Start over

and serve!

!

Ecclesiastes 1:9

*"What has been will be again,
what has been done will be done again;
there is nothing new under the sun."*

*Caution and forewarning:
Before you begin reading this book, please prepare
your mind to see your life and our
world in a new light.*

1
CHRISTIAN REVIVAL DIET™

"It is for freedom that Christ has set us free. Stand firm, then, and do not let yourselves be burdened again by a yoke of slavery." **Galatians 5:1**

"For God did not send His Son into the world to condemn the world, but to save the world through Him." **John 3:17**

The Christian Revival Diet™ is a simple way to help you on the path that God wants to lead you on with the goal of transformation in all areas of your life.

But why another diet book? There are too many out there you might say. You are correct! There are way too many out there, however I see a gap in most of these books as they don't relate to the Biblical foundation for complete nourishment, and with the state of our world we need to have a strong foundation in Christ and more behind the 'why' versus the 'how'.

The world has so many people captive and in slavery to sin and unhealthy living and so many books out there which only complicate the issue and end up making things worse by treating the symptoms rather than looking at the root causes.

The Christian Revival Diet™ strives to focus on the foundation of healthy living concepts while striving to live a more Biblically-strong Christian lifestyle.

If any of these phrases define or describe your current condition, this book can help you:

I'm forgetful

I don't follow through on things

I feel like I'm not as active as I once was

I eat for comfort and not for nutrition

I exercise sporadically

I am moody and emotional

I have strange habits and neurosis

I judge others

I gossip

I feel inadequate in some areas of my life

I'm not confident in my abilities

I don't know what I want to do with my life

I find it difficult to stay organized

I find myself eating impulsively or when I'm not even really hungry

I'm on medication for diet-related ailments

I don't feel as healthy as I once did

I find it hard to wake up in the morning

I don't know what recipes to cook or what to order in a restaurant

Packaged foods are the only thing I can cook

I don't know which foods are healthy

I feel too busy to make effective choices

I've tried package diets and they work for a while and then I return to the same lifestyle as before, and the weight comes back.

I binge eat now and then

I don't eat healthy proportions

I ache and have pains where I didn't before

I don't feel satisfied in many areas of my life

I eat more than I should

I may have a sugar addiction

I crave things and never feel full

I don't even know what righteous living is

I'm reckless and not as planned out as I want to be

I suffer from sleeplessness or I sleep too much

I have a hard time controlling my behavior (words, food, actions)

I would like to get more organized

I have a hard time following through

Some people think I'm manic

I've started diets or resolutions only to fail or retreat to same routines rapidly after I make progress.

There are too many books with empty messages and hard-to-interpret directions, expensive and time consuming recipes and rigid, hard-to-follow rules. These jaded and counterfeit messages myopically encourage us to stumble through our daily choices. The reality of the lives we live in a world that overflows with empty distractions, shallow busy-ness, empty nutrition, empty calories, and empty messages while we search for joy that leaves us feeling more empty or only with limited satisfaction for the moment.

This book is only for those who want revival, renewal, redirection and a new lens to look through at the world. They want fresh invigorated eyes with a lasting solution, not just a quick fix. The commitment and dedication takes work nevertheless may even be easier than you think. However it still takes discipline and commitment. This book is for those who want change in all aspects of their lives, spiritually, mentally, emotionally, physically, relationally, and more.

This book is only for a person who truly wants to think through decisions and make a conscious effort to affect change in their life and the lives of those around them. They are not content with the outcome of mediocrity. They crave success and want to live in the light of Christ's love and blessing, no matter the circumstances.

The Christian Revival Diet™ is only for people who want the truth and continue down a path to seek it. They realize that it's not going to happen in '5 days to lose 10lbs', 'eat only something' or 'some other gimmicky moniker' trendy book.

This book isn't written for a quick fix, this book is for sustained action.

The Christian Revival Diet™ is an awakening of all aspects of your life, i.e. (emotionally, physically, financially, relationally, spiritually, nutritionally, and so much more.) You must be someone earnestly seeking to hear the truth and the take action. Before I describe what the major premise is, let me tell you about why and how the inspiration for this book came to be.

I am not an author by nature or by countenance. I am only writing this because the message needs to be communicated. So please pardon any crazy syntax or grammar errors. Please look for the main message and most importantly the application for your life.

My passion in life has been towards the financial side as an economist. I am always striving to make the most of time, relationships, thrift, money and value. I am a financial guy who wants to live a healthier life and apply the principles of maximized and optimized finances, living, and health to the fullest in all areas.

My personal journey and the application of the Christian Revival Diet™ begins:

Here was my issue and my stumbling block....I was a 21 year old, 6 pack abs and in shape guy with my weight hovering between 164 and 172, and then came the professional world and raising children. By age 34, I was between 172 and 177. I was still able to run well, mountain bike, play hockey and soccer and enjoy a fairly active lifestyle. I know that everyone warns "your metabolism might start slowing down" as a nice way of giving some cautionary warning.

Nevertheless, once my parents said, "David is really filling out", it sounded more like an "age based rite of passage and an excuse for overweight aging in the United States".

From ages 34-40, it seemed all my friends and business

colleagues wanted to meet for breakfast, lunch, coffee or something surrounding to food or drink. This led us to discussions about "saving the world" or "pains of the world" while we filled our stomachs and achieved greater levels of sedentary living and piled on excess weight. Instead of wanting to go for a run or a bike ride or to do some fun activity outside together, we became café cowboys.

Effortlessly and slowly the weight continued creeping until it really hit me came at age 40. I was invited to take part in an office sponsored weight loss contest, because the coordinator thought that it'd be easy for her to lose more weight than me. As she thought that I didn't have much weight to lose, I hid it and was still fairly average for a Midwestern man in mid-life.

I chuckled and thought that I didn't have much to lose. The reality was when I weighed myself for the initial weigh in and I weighed 194. That is about 32 pounds over my age weight at age 21. Indeed I had filled out quite nicely. However, if that was filling out, why didn't I feel better? As it stood compared to so many other "filled-out-middle-aged-monkeys", I was still slimmer than most of my peers, even by Body Mass Index (BMI) standards.

Embarrassingly, no one told me what the effects the "filling-out creep" would have on my body. I began was beginning to notice the negative side effects of this slow weight gain.

I started feeling aches in my knees and back on some of my runs. I never had these types of aches before. I'd run 6-10 miles on a Saturday night come home, and complain to my wife, saying "it sucks getting old with all these new found aches." As my knees would feel on shorter runs tight and stressed. The sad reality is that nobody told me the truth of my new-found body…. 30 pounds overweight.

"One who is full loathes honey from the comb, but to the hungry even what is bitter tastes sweet." Proverbs 27:7

If the above proverb was written today when there are many synthetic sweeteners perhaps the proverb would read, *"One who eats unhealthy junk food, will only become insatiably hungry and eventually grow weak, fat, dumb, dependent and captive to disease."*

If I eat some sprouts, broccoli, spinach or something, I feel full and happy over the long run. However, if I throw in something with high fructose corn syrup or lots of sugar, I only crave more. Reading a research article about dopamine, I was surprised to learn some intriguing insights of how it relates to your brain and life.

Dopamine is a neurochemical that regulates motivation, pleasure, and on the negative in extreme cases it can create pleasure seeking addicts. After eating a bite of milk chocolate, dopamine is sent to your brain and transmits to the rest of your body. *"Ahh, that chocolate is good, eat more of it... don't stop now."*

Like any person who starts recreational feeding the pleasure seeking part of their brain, basically feeding their craving, they lose self-control. If this is left unchecked it could potentially create an addiction. Sugar is probably the most dangerous thing that tempts us daily.

The challenge with junk food is that it's readily available, and very low cost and easy to prepare, and offers many of the same quick pleasure fulfilling rewards. You can drive while using it, use it and keep your job, and go pretty much anywhere and get it.

The greatest challenge is that your dopamine receptors develop a tolerance of the sugar; they become calloused and what used to give your body that same message of pleasure and satiation now takes significantly more amount of chocolate to achieve.

The intestinal tract, however, searches for nutrients that your body requires; fiber, vitamins, minerals, fats, carbohydrates, and such. It doesn't know at all what you put in your mouth as a food item = like spinach per se, the intestinal tract can't really taste. It works on your behalf to take in nutrients and transfer those your body needs to help run it and what it can't digest will be excreted or stored as fat because it gets overloaded. Thank God that your intestinal tract is forgiving most of the time.

How does our intestinal tract honor God?

Isn't it fascinating how God made your mouth to taste and long for pleasure (be that sweet, sour, bitter, crispy, crunchy, spicy, etc.) and your intestinal tract completely void of taste sensations. Imagine if your taste buds acted from your intestinal tract. You'd only eat what worked in harmony to truly fill you to a proper nutrient level, completely full and energetic for the journey. Just think of how the food industry would have to change to accommodate to your intestinal tract needs.

When I lived in Japan, I was so eager to share some of my favorite sweets with the Japanese students. I requested my parents to send me some red licorice and some bite-sized candy bars individually wrapped so they could taste these wonderful pieces of "American traditional candy bars"; a common staple and symbol of our culture just like popcorn, hotdogs, ice cream and apple pie.

I received the package and opened it eagerly. Since I had not enjoyed any of these items for about six months, I was salivating even before I opened the package.

I opened one of the candy bars and popped it in my mouth and then grabbed another rapidly. It didn't taste like I had remembered it. It was more synthetic tasting and kind of chemically, waxy, over-sweet. I ignored that feeling and focused on the mental buzz from the perceived sugar rush of joy entering my mind and mouth.

The next day, I handed out samples to more than 180 students over the course of the 6 classes, and all except one of the students said "Amai" which means in Japanese "sweet".

I nodded to myself like a dope dealer, thinking *yes, little boys and girls, it is super sweet and isn't that great'*. I thought the word 'sweet' they were using was a good thing, as that'd be how we American's view our desserts and drinks in this country and typically use the word. The sweeter in many cases the better.

But then I realized the students hadn't even finished the treats I had so proudly shared. In most cases, it was completely hard to view that there was even a nibble on the bars. Although they thanked me politely, most didn't even consume what I gave them.

Upon further surveying the trash receptacle, in typical Japanese style, most of the wrappers were even rewrapped nicely around candy bars.

After this happened after all six of my classes I wondered how their taste buds could be so different than mine? Dopamine receptors was the answer. Our receptors are like calloused addicts, where theirs are like timid young freshman. While living in Japan, I enjoyed many of the traditional Japanese sweets, they were much more mild and healthy tasting. Many times the balance of protein and carbohydrates, like some of their bean, sesame seed and rice type desserts, were actually quite healthy.

Pancakes! Everybody loves pancakes with Maple syrup, I thought. My wife and I taught a cooking class with a typical pancake breakfast. For one of the schools making them some nice fluffy pancakes another time. I seriously had the naivety to think that I was bringing in some revolutionary new food sensation to their palate. The results were the same with most of the items being dumped in the trash. The same result from my earlier candy scenario = with the same type of result as the chocolate and licorice.

Frankly, that is where most of the food we can buy would have the greatest benefit = in the trash.

After two years of living there, my calloused dopamine

receptors softened from the harsh extremes of my American diet away from our sugary levels.

Some of you Japanese culture aficionados, you might question, that you have seen some of the Japanese packaged sweets and they do dabble in some interesting and rich junk foods that are similar to ours. Mind you, I was in the rural country side where many of the items were hand made, and not industrially fabricated. When I visited the larger cities, many of the foods I saw did lead more towards the fabricated packaged sweeter versions similar to my western tastes. But none that seemed to rival our levels of high fructose corn syrup and sugar shock to the taste buds.

Our food scientists have mastered the achievement of creating highly addictive, intensely sweet, salty, fatty foods for good reason. We love them (at least our minds love the feelings we get from them, our intestinal tract doesn't love them). We can't get enough, and the companies sell a lot more of them and make huge profit margins as well. It's so difficult as willpower, philosophy, positive mantras, your mom telling you not too eat some of these temptations, are no match for the highly addictive items that are sold en masse almost everywhere you look.

Imagine what our grocery stores would look like if there was only non-processed healthy foods. That is why I enjoy going on backpacking trips where I am removed from the ability to shop. There is no possibility to make any impulse purchases, and I pack for energy, efficiency and nutrients.

There is such a peace in the nature about not being bombarded by vending machines around every corner, drive-thrus with signs offering fries, shakes and burgers, fast food on every corner, and at every register and at stores you would typically have not considered in the junk food business.

About 8 years ago, I thought I'd give a big box home improvement store a suggestion that they could sell soda and candy at the registers, as a regional store near us does that.

While I was remodeling our house, I thought it would be nice to grab a candy bar or a stick of beef jerky.

My selfish motivation was so that I could walk from my house to the large home improvement warehouse and not have to go to the grocery store as well to get a snack. As a married couple without kids, our refrigerator was often empty as we went out to eat so much. I wanted to get the supplies for the next part of a home project and grab a quick snack as well.

Sadly, they took the suggestion, and added more food items to their check-out lanes. Now temptation looms at another location, from big box warehouse stores and virtually wherever you look. Hey junk food sells. It's the legalized addiction that goes on silently in our modern era.

Are you going with the flow unthinkingly? Are you a person who feels you are in the norm of your culture? What does your cultural eating habits look like?

_____

_____

_____

_____

All of the Japanese students were steadfast in their approach: Politely threw the junk food away while still showing gracious appreciation.

If the shoe were on the other foot and they brought some sweetened anchovies with almonds (a salty, crunchy savory snack that many Japanese enjoy), do you think our American students would have been polite and just thrown it away? I think not. I think they would have made a scene and been super direct in their dislike for it.

Coming back to my weight loss needs…. I pondered these questions.

But why didn't anyone say it to me? Did they think I wouldn't listen? It might have reduced my life expectancy a few years, added to future medical costs, limited my ability to be engaged in my children or grandchildren's lives. So why were people so complacently nice to me and not more honest?

In all relationships and situations, we have three things we can communicate, and all are correct at various times and scenarios. Wisdom comes from knowing the tactful time and place to speak your concerns about the item or take the appropriate action or inaction based on where you sense God is leading you in your specific circumstance.

Confront: Speaking truth into someone's life is to show them a facet of the diamond they often times can't see. When the person is ready to listen then it is such a blessing of care and love.

Proverbs 16:13 speaks to the focus that *"Kings take pleasure in honest lips; they value the one who speaks what is right."*

Have you confronted issues when it's been appropriate? Do you know someone who had unhealthy habits that would benefit from your communication to them?

_____

_____

_____

_____

_____

Avoid: When we avoid, we end up making our life a bit easier for us. However, we may not make their lives better, as we disregard what they may need by hearing truth. We may avoid the person, the topic, or the situation.

"Mockers resent correction, so they avoid the wise." Proverbs 15:12

Have you avoided the correct things or circumstances in your life or another person that you have connected with? Where could you grow in this area?

_____

_____

_____

_____

Tolerate: When we decide to tolerate some situation we in essence are approving it. When we tolerate our own sins or the sins of someone else, we basically are accepting the sin as ok. Even if someone doesn't ask us to forgive them for something they've done wrong, we should still forgive them as that is what we are called to do.

Just as on the cross dying, Christ said, Father forgive them for they know not what they do. I do believe that we should be tolerant when someone repents, confesses and seeks to strive to request forgiveness.

The challenge with this is that if we do not point out a sin or help another see the area of growth needed, our actions or inactions are guilty of helping their sin or what we have left undone and what we could have done to support their salvation or need.

If you see a child about to run across the street where a car is coming. Would you tolerate it thinking, "Oh they can do whatever they want?" Or would you avoid it by turning your back, and saying under your breath, "people do things for their reasons."

I hope you would confront it by yelling, "come here now as fast as you can, get out of the street."

It makes me see that when danger or sin is threatening someone our role is to graciously point it out to the other person. I know that we can't force anyone to eat or not eat anything.

"Be tolerant with one another and forgive one another whenever any of you has a complaint against someone else. You must forgive one another just as the Lord has forgiven you." Colossians 3:13

Has your tolerance been appropriate in reviewing situations where someone may be in jeopardy?

_____

_____

_____

_____

I believe it's not selfish to speak the truth, if the motivations and intentions are in check. The individual you are speaking with as well needs to be open. You must check your emotions however, as sometimes holding back for your reasons of being liked, not offending someone, or not getting into a confrontation may actually be a form of selfishness that is as well not very honoring to Christ. Jesus called us to be salt and light, not maple syrup and peppermint patties.

Even my physician, when asked about my aches, said, "age'll do it to you".

I spent 3 visits, and probably more than thirty tests, and the physician said to me "you are in optimal health". Looking back on it, 'optimal health', was his diagnosis and a dangerous one at that; 'optimal health' for what? And compared to what? I should have asked?

I can't fault my doctor, and while I think he could have done a better job, the ownership falls 100% on me. I could look in the mirror and see that there was less definition in my abs than before. Instead of a 6 pack abs it was a softer contoured two or four pack abs, depending on the light. If you would have compared my body fat percentages to other American's I would have still ranged in the top 10-25% of in the healthy range. But why then did I feel so lousy, achy and not in shape?

I had to own the responsibility. I had to own the phrase *'you sleep in the body you make'*.

The reality is that over 20 years, every day's seemingly benign choices led eventually to the current state of my reality. A handful of chocolate here, an extra bananas foster desert after the steak meal at the restaurant, a few late night snacks, and another skipped workout session and just like that, my new nickname could have been "marshmallow". I was at least 30 pounds over my optimum weight.

Thanks to supportive prayer requests and God's sovereignty, and after many nights praying to God for direction, counting calories, exercising, reducing junk foods, sleeping more and by His grace and direction finally just saying, "No more excuses" and "I'm going to regain the edge I had when I was @ age 21!". I even contacted my doctor's office from my youth that had my physical from that age and that became my mission and my focus to hit that weight.

Well two plus years later I achieved my goal. I won the contest by losing 35 pounds over 4 months and maintained it steadily since then.

Now, praise the Lord, I am back to my target weight and my abs are have greater definition once again, and I'm able to run for three to four hours without any aches or pains, play ice hockey with my kids for one to two hours now nearing age 43.

Praise God! I am closer to optimal health than I was two years earlier and my parents have commented that I look in better shape than when I was 21 with better muscle tone! Praise God as I've held pretty consistent for weight +/- 2.7 lbs for two years hovering at about 162.

For me this has been a true revival and awakening in my life, and now as God opened this door, there have been so many more other doors opening, as I continue to pray to God for wisdom and direction in my life.

This journey is teaching me how to be a better Christian, a better father, husband, dad and son while living out the Christian Revival needed in our land.

That is also my prayer for you as you hear some of the insights from my experience, and you discern what path you will choose and, most importantly, you allow God to lead you through the path of your own understanding. Remember He is sovereign!

The major premise and simple path of this diet is one focus:

Honoring Christ

By

Committing to God's direction in your life

Through

Ingesting a healthy balanced diet of God's word, God's food, God's direction, God's healthy living and God's rest in your life and living for Him in all things.

And as a financial guy, I'm always into math formulas to illustrate the point. Simply put, here is the equation:

Your life is currently defined and created by this:
Current Reality = A + B + C + D + E + ...

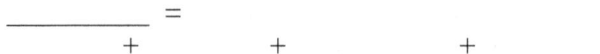

Your revived life that you are striving for has a desired outcome. The simple equation is to reconstruct the items that make your current reality by the outcomes that will get you to your desired life.

Desired Life = G + O + D

_____ = _____ + _____ + _____

Remember Matthew 7:7 *"Ask and it will be given to you; seek and you will find; knock and the door will be opened to you."* The bottom line is that you need to ask, and God will give it to you, the reality it may not be in your timing, but that being said it doesn't mean we shouldn't ask now with expectation.

What are you asking for?

_____

_____

_____

_____

_____

What do you think God wants you to do?

_____

_____

_____

_____

On a scale of one to ten, 1 being not at all and 10 being earnestly with all your heart striving, please list your level of diligence and direction that you are striving towards:

_____

_____

_____

_____

_____

I wish it was more complicated than this and I know our human tendencies are to try to complicate this with limited success. The negative self-talk in your mind may even say something like. *"I don't need an equation, philosophy, or even God. I just want what I'm supposed to eat, do, and say and then everything will be easier."*

Let's look at the definition of the word "re"

a prefix, occurring orig. in loanwords from Latin, used to form verbs denoting **action in a backward direction** *(recede; return; revert), action in answer to or intended to undo a situation (rebel; remove; respond; restore; revoke), or action done over, often with the implication that the outcome of the original action was in some way impermanent or inadequate, or that the performance of the new action brings back an earlier state of affairs (recapture; reoccur; repossess; retype; revitalize, reenergize)*

Definition from : Random House Kernerman Webster's College Dictionary, © 2010 K Dictionaries Ltd. Copyright 2005, 1997, 1991 by Random House, Inc. All rights reserved.

What a great concept, to "re"turn something to its original state or action. While the definition "re" in the above definition relates to the action of going in a backward direction and that's the general feel. I'd encourage your focus be toward looking forward as you prepare for an eternity with Christ.

God created you in His image, and Adam (man) and Eve's (woman's) choice in the garden got us kicked out to have a limited time-bound life on earth with our earthly bodies having a planned obsolescence (failure rate).

This body of ours will turn back to dust. Based on God's call and our response, eternal hell or eternal heaven eventually will be our place of residence. Let me stress the focus living with eternity in mind.

If you died tomorrow what would you write on the back of this business card for your newborn son? Go ahead write it down:

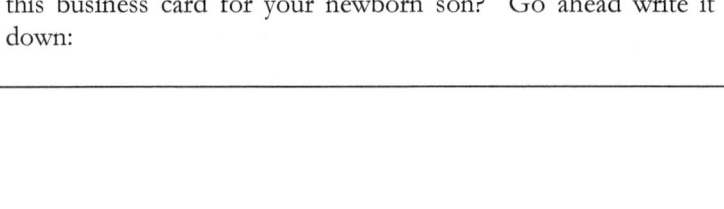

A pretty serious question asked to me from a gentleman I only had met once before. He was an owner and president of many successful companies. The gentleman's net worth was most likely well in the billions, and he was a gentle yet focused and determined man with eyes like eagles, watching every move you make, and a calm demeanor.

Considering his prominence in the business community as well as his wealth, and the fact that I was sitting on a pretty nice leather couch his house overlooking Lake Minnetonka from the quaint town of Woodland, I was a bit intimidated. I sat down with him, as an impressionable 35 year old, as he invited me to his house for lunch with a friend.

That was the first question he asked. "If you died tomorrow what would you write on the back of this business card for your newborn son? Go ahead write it down:" (he knew I had a newborn son of less than one, so I think he phrases it differently depending on what he thinks your heart is)

It definitely made me sweat. Since he was a client of ours, I wanted to make a favorable impression. After a quick moment I wrote on the back of the card:

"Jesus loves you and so do I; Trust God and read your Bible"

He then asked me to write that down with today's date in his book of quotes from other people he has met. As I started writing he stood up and leaned closer to me, "Are you sure that is what you would write?" Somewhat testing my resolve and belief.

I wasn't the only one he asked that question to. He had hundreds of people who had written things into that book of his. He was a man who sought to see into the window of your soul, really into the true you. After I wrote it down, he asked "Why?"

Later we spoke for about five hours about faith, church choices, understanding life as well as family and kids. Everything he said had meaning and was focused. He dove to the core of the subjects rapidly and stayed focused on engaging conversation like no one I have ever met before.

The thoughts of why I would write that as the most important words, I could give my newborn son came to me as I did a fast prayer and discern what legacy I would like to leave my son and the children yet to come. I thought about teaching them all I had learned, how to live, relate, connect, work, care for others, etc. But in the end it was a quick understanding that the greatest source of wisdom I could ever hope for them to search out was that of God's love and the words within the Bible.

It was a sobering relief as I wrote that and God gave me the strength to stand firm on my resolve, but those four hours went by rapidly, as he machined gunned questions non-stop at me about many matters. He barely gave me time to reflect.

I had been warned about him from some others who knew him that he was, as they called him, "quite a bit eccentric". I personally was relieved at the truth, sincerity and open inquisitive nature of his quest and zest for getting to know people deeply. The conversation with him was much more meaningful than the superficial conversations I've had with other people.

At the end of the conversation he mentioned to me that I sure gave him quite a lot of things to think about, and that he needed to have a bit of a rest to consider some of these items.

His first wife had passed away more than 10 years prior from cancer, and it left him with a lot of unanswered questions and frustrations about life and his place in it.

Looking back now, I tried to role model my faith and speak of my faith, but I never asked him if he would receive Christ in his heart, give his life to Jesus, repent of his sins and turn from them.

Honestly I was in fear of asking that for my own selfish reasons and stayed on the motto "most people won't read the Bible, but if you claim to be a Christian they read your life". While this is a contemporary saying, and I value the role modeling influence one has and actions are greater than words, based on this scenario I wish I had asked the tough question and not wimped out.

The reality is that if any person tries to "read" another person's life they are going to be able to find flaws. That is the nature of living in the fallen world. No organization, no pastor, no Pope, no church, no ministry is without sin in this fallen world. Yes, some may sin less than others, but there is no one, not one, who at this moment in time lives on the earth that isn't flawed.

We are so trapped in the sinfulness of this world only through God's grace can we even get a rare glimpse of his vastness, mightiness and holiness.

One year after that intense conversation the gentleman passed away. I hadn't seen him between our meeting and the time of his passing. I'm not sure if he personally accepted Jesus as his savior, and if my inaction aided to his eternity being spent in hell. I can only ask Christ for forgiveness for my selfish inaction and what I left undone of not being as direct as I now looking back know I should have been. I only pray that my words and actions did potentially have an influence on his life.

Jesus says in Matthew 6:9-13:

"Our Father in heaven, hallowed be your name, your kingdom come, your will be done, on earth as it is in heaven. Give us today our daily bread. And forgive us our debts, as we also have forgiven our debtors. And lead us not into temptation, but deliver us from the evil one."

The evil one is not to be underestimated. Satan rules this world and he broke Adam and Eve's resolve in the Garden of Eden. If you think you are not one step away from Satan claiming victory over you, you are already in his grasp.

As a child growing up at an Episcopal Church we used to recite this prayer. Although as a child I didn't fully listen or take to heart the meaning or the application and implication for my life. I wanted to highlight some of the Biblical basis for this prayer, and let you see how it applies to your life.

"Most merciful God, we confess that we have sinned against you in thought, word, and deed, by what we have done, and by what we have left undone. We have not loved you with our whole heart; we have not loved our neighbors as ourselves. We are truly sorry and we humbly repent, for the sake of your Son Jesus Christ, have mercy on us and forgive us; that we may delight in your will, and walk in your ways, to the glory of your Name. Amen."

Episcopal *Book of Common Prayer*

"Most Merciful God we confess that we have sinned against you in thought, word, and deed,"

Biblical references to the above:
Romans 3:23 *"All have sinned and fall short of the glory of God."*

1 John 1:10 *"If we claim we have not sinned, we make him out to be a liar and His truth word is not in us."*

"...by what we have done, and by what we have left undone."

Biblical reference to the above quote:

Romans 7:14-25 *"We know that the law is spiritual; but I am unspiritual, sold as a slave to sin. I do not understand what I do. For what I want to do I do not do, but what I hate I do. And if I do what I do not want to do, I agree that the law is good. As it is, it is no longer I myself who do it, but it is sin living in me. For I know that good itself does not dwell in me, that is, in my sinful nature. For I have the desire to do what is good, but I cannot carry it out. For I do not do the good I want to do, but the evil I do not want to do - this I keep on doing. Now if I do what I do not want to do, it is no longer I who do it, but it is sin living in me that does it. So I find this law at work: Although I want to do good, evil is right there with me. For in my inner being I delight in God's law; but I see another law at work in me, waging war against the law of my mind and making me a prisoner of the law of sin at work within me.*

What a wretched man I am! Who will rescue me from this body that is subject to death? Thanks be to God, who delivers me through Jesus Christ our Lord!

So then, I myself in my mind am a slave to God's law, but in my sinful nature a slave to the law of sin. "

Wow! So much to think about, so much that convicts our sinful nature, and so much to grow from. Whenever I hear or say the phrase, *"Forgive us for what we have left undone",* I always feel even more convicted. Especially with the notion that I know what I have done, but it convicts me in the matter of what I haven't been aware of to do, missed out doing, or completely avoided altogether. It shows me the willful ignorance or unintentional items that I could have affected but didn't.

What do we leave undone? The greatest thing we leave undone is not asking people if they have asked Christ personally to live in their hearts, forgive them of their sins and repent, confess and turn from their wicked and evil ways. But there are other things in our life that we could have done for Christ we didn't do. This convicts me and makes me want to be more attentive to the opportunities that avail themselves to me to stand firm for Christ.

Is there something in your life that you have left undone?

_____

_____

_____

_____

What do you think Jesus would like you to do about it?

_____

_____

_____

"...*We have not loved you with our whole heart; we have not loved our neighbors as ourselves.*"

Biblical reference to the above:

>Matthew 22:34-40
>*"Hearing that Jesus had silenced the Sadducees, the Pharisees got together. One of them, an expert in the law, tested Him with this question: 'Teacher, which is the greatest commandment in the Law?' Jesus replied: 'Love the Lord your God with all your heart and with all your soul and with all your mind.' This is the first and greatest commandment. And the second is like it: 'Love your neighbor as yourself'. All the Law and the Prophets hand on these two commandments."*

"...*We are truly sorry and we humbly repent, for the sake of your Son Jesus Christ, have mercy on us and forgive us;*"

Biblical references to the above:
>Matthew 6:12
>*"And forgive us our debts, as we also have forgiven our debtors."*

Luke 11:4
"Forgive us our sins, for we also forgive everyone who sins against us. And lead us not into temptation."

Luke 11:4
"If we confess our sins, He is faithful and just and will forgive us our sins and purify us from all unrighteousness."

"...that we may delight in your will, and walk in your ways, to the glory of your Name. Amen"

Biblical reference to the above:

Proverbs 9:6
"Leave your simple ways and you will live; walk in the way of insight."

Malachi 3:12
"Then all the nations will call you blessed, for yours will be a delightful land."

Revelation 4:11
"You are worthy, our Lord and God, to receive glory and honor and power, for you created all things, and by your will they were created and have their being."

What would you write to your children on the back of a business card if you knew that was the last message you were going to leave them?

Is your life a 100% projection of that message that they will remember you for?

_____

_____

_____

_____

What in your life can you better work on to show your children that message in how you live?

_____

_____

_____

_____

Many churches stray from the altar call or asking for a commitment to follow Christ. A study by the Barna group (source internet) found that only 45% of Christians who claim to follow Christ have been born again. In John 3:3, it states that we must be born again to see the kingdom of heaven.

If we ask Jesus to forgive our sins and choose to follow him, we will be given a heavenly eternal existence. That is the promise He gives to us.

Consider that the only real focus should be on our preparation for an eternity in either Heaven or Hell.

What is 100 years compared to 100,000,000,000,000,000,000,000,000,000,000 to the 'infinity'th power? That might be more stars than in the universe!

I personally would encourage you to follow Christ and declare your need for him, repent of your sins, and turn from your sins to Jesus. As my understanding of Heaven is much more desirable than the alternative.

As we are forward moving human beings, stuck on our time bound escalator moving us forward and faster indeed, the greatest thing about the past is that it is over, and the greatest thing about the present is to live for God in the moment and the future is that we don't know what it will be, but God gives us the opportunity to remember the hope only He gives us.

If you were to pack your suitcase for an eternal trip, what would you pack today? How would you prepare? What would you want to retain in your mind to bring with you?

What would you'd pack for eternity?

_____

_____

_____

_____

_____

What sins do you need to repent or turn away from? Do you have a right relationship with Christ in order to have Him be your source and strength to guide you away from your sin?

_____

_____

_____

_____

How many people have you heard speaking about "When I was younger, I used to do this?" or "Now that I'm older I can do that." We all wish we were younger. We can wish wrinkles away, pains to subside, or strength to return or wish we could run and not grow tired like when we were youthful, but the inevitable will happen.

God made the gift of aging and death for a reason. That is the conclusion to His desire, with the goal of planting for us a longing to know Him more and live our life for His glory. But we don't have to be living in a body that is neglected or shown little respect over our years.

I'd encourage you to think of this book as a reminder and a call to proceed forward in a direction to begin anew the vitality that God has given us, with a goal of honoring Him to help our service for Him during our short time here.

What life does God have for you? What is holding you back?

_____

_____

_____

_____

Whatever your life goal may be: to lose weight, look better, feel better, gain an athletic edge, perform better, rest better, or serve wherever you are to your utmost, by God's power, this book may be a springboard for you.

In the past ten years I've literally read hundreds of books about the above items, and some have very good points. However, more important than any of the books, has been the emphasis on implementing the changes and acting upon the results.

I've weighed myself in the morning when I wake up and every evening when I go to bed to make sure that I'm on track with my goals. We'll highlight some of the other things that I have implemented throughout the process. Your journey may have similarities. However I am 100% confident it will be completely different with its own set of challenges, opportunities, and consequences. Praise God!

I know not one person who couldn't live a little bit better in some way. How about you?

Living for Christ is all about perspective and valuing it from whichever vantage point you are seeing things. The real perspective comes through our will to intertwine Christ's direction in all aspects of our lives. So, as we strive to seek His will for us, remember that on this side of heaven we can never fully grasp His infinite and omnificent will.

Please consider the ideas, stories or vantage points limited to the extent that I am in the sinful system as you are and even within God's will there are times when His will is played out completely different than another's, but all the while still in His will. I've heard people say that you are only in control of your controllables, however I think as the book continues you will see that you are in total control of your controllables and God has a plan nonetheless and is in total control even with you going the direction you freely want to go.

If you are a person who only wants to see things one way, please don't read this book. I suggest you read a book like the 'cabbage only diet' (if there is such a book) or some other type of catchy trendy bestseller. If you want statistics, scientific justification, and fancy recipes there are many books that focus on this area. There are benefits in all of these items as they can give you better knowledge of certain nutritional values. The Christian Revival Diet™ however is different.

The refreshing focus of the Christian Revival Diet™ is that it is a philosophy and an applied lifestyle that you can live by. Some could even call it a lens through which to view the world as you make choices that either honor God or detract from His will.

I've sought to seek Biblical justification and rationale as the foundation of this book.

The goal is to give you thoughtful considerations to make better decisions when faced with choices and live a life worthy of Christ's blessing. Wouldn't it be great, if upon arrival in heaven, God said to you *"Well done, good and faithful servant."* Matthew 25:21

The Christian Revival Diet™ starts with nutrition at the core, but my prayer is that you will see the transferrable application and cross pollination that will flow into other areas of your life, professionally and personally. (Not only physically)

Our nation, and much of our world, is for the most part spiritually, morally, nutritionally, and financially bankrupt. The current state of affairs in our country and our world dictates that we need a revival in our nutritional approach to what we consume.

As the definition of revival from *Collins English Dictionary* © *2013* says that it's a reawakening of faith or renewal of commitment to a religion. If a revival is needed, then that assumes that we have fallen away or rebelled. The truth is that God has NOT changed. We have as people, as a nation, as a society. We need to return to Christ's truth and revive this land, repent of our sins, and turn to Him in all things.

One of the most common things we end up doing, without thinking, is eating. Our reasons are not thought out, especially in more affluent and wealthy societies. We eat for pleasure, taste, boredom, social gatherings, energy, social entertainment, etc. We eat and don't often question what it is we are eating. We rarely question the colors, the preparation, the ingredients, the source, the contents and the concoctions that we trust will fuel us. We often trust blindly that if someone sells it to us, it must be quality.

Many of us are fat, lazy, content and diseased. We eat and are never full. I love in Proverbs 27 as a whole, but specifically Proverbs 27:19-20 *"As water reflects the face, so one's life reflects the heart. Death and destruction are never satisfied, and neither are human eyes."*

If a reawakened interest in what we consume (audibly, orally, visually, mentally) occurs, which I believe has started in some areas, I'm convinced that with the proper perspective it will help birth a much greater revival in many areas of our troubled world. That is why I have written this book.

Just as sin can literally "sear" our conscience which in turn, like a callous, challenges our sensitivity to things which we should not see, hear, taste, think, speak, associate with, etc. Do you think our nation has a seared conscience? Do you clearly know what sin is? Understanding sin helps us to know it, avoid it, confess it, and to be successful as standing with Christ under it.

As 1 Corinthians 6:12-13 says *"So, if you think you are standing firm, be careful that you don't fall! No temptation has overtaken you except what is common to mankind. And God is faithful; he will not let you be tempted beyond what you can bear. But when you are tempted, he will also provide a way out so that you can endure it."*

Indeed, yes, it is truly so that you can endure and find a way out from the temptation or the trial that you may are facing or that you will face.

1 Timothy 4:1-2 *"The Spirit clearly says that in later times some will abandon the faith and follow deceiving spirits and things taught by demons. Such teachings come through hypocritical liars, whose consciences have been seared as with a hot iron."*

Everyone is seared by sin to a certain level (just like our dopamine receptors). Only Christ can heal us, but that scar tissue remains as a memory to our conscious of the need for humility and grace in light of our own sinful reality.

What areas do you think you might be "seared" or "overly-calloused" in your life or the world around you?

_____

_____

_____

_____

What are you waiting for?

_____

_____

_____

_____

How we live in all aspects reflects what we believe in, so how are you living? (For better or for worse)

_____

_____

_____

_____

If Jesus were sitting next to you, what would He say about what you are doing?

_____

_____

_____

A revival has historically been preceded by times of tragedy, darkness, loss, and sorrow. It's sad but true that we only turn to Jesus at times we are broken or severely challenged. Unfortunately or fortunately, this is dismal state of affairs in so many aspects of our contemporary living.

Just look around. Do you think a revival is needed?

The opposite to revival would be devival.

I thought I made this word up since I've never heard it before, but then when I looked it up online, I discovered that devival is a 'return to the worldly pleasures of the day'. Well how fitting is that! Someone beat me to claiming that word.

If you don't see physically overweight people, or see physically malnourished people or spiritually malnourished souls, longing for so much more, then you may be one of them, as you think what you see is normal around you.

In the areas of nutrition, fitness and health, many people in our nation have come to a point of willful ignorance. Blindly stuck in their sin, and a sort of collective laziness, they often make other centered excuses and recline in complacent comfort living in their bad habits. Or on the contrary they have become excessive and come to a point of over training and idolizing their workouts and regimens. It's hard to find balance.

God's word puts life's questions in the right perspective.

1 Timothy 4:6-10 speaks about the importance of physical training with a greater emphasis on spiritual training. This must be at the center of our life.

"If you point these things out to brothers and sisters, you will be a good minister of Christ Jesus, nourished on the truths of the faith and of the good teaching that you have followed. Have nothing to do with godless myths and old wives' tales; rather train yourself to be godly. For physical training is of some value, but godliness has value for all things, holding promise for both the present life and the life to come. This is a trustworthy saying that deserves full acceptance. That is why we labor and strive, because we have put our hope in the living God, who is the Savior of all people, and especially of those who believe." 1 Timothy 4:6-10

My father sat me down when I was about 16 or 17 years old during a rebellious stage of my youth, and said to me, "Someday you will have to look yourself in the mirror and answer the question, *'Am I pleased with what I see?' 'Did I do what I was meant to with my time here?"*

When reflecting on that it leads me to the reality that as a kid when I didn't want to really see what I was or what I was doing, I would just simply avoid the mirror. Avoidance. It's a form of self-denial and other rationalization (or a form of scapegoating).

In light of that and the obvious rebellion I would try to find substantiation and justification for my lack of right living.

We do know that Christ will judge everyone. As it says in Revelation 22:12, *"Look, I am coming soon! My reward is with me, and I will give to each person according to what they have done"*.

God judges. The reflection you look at in the mirror will not be the face you see when you enter heaven and see face the Almighty. You will see Christ and He will not judge your rationalization.

If you are in a state of complacent denial, willful ignorance or just don't want to own up to the responsibility of looking at yourself in the mirror. Don't fret or get down on yourself, it's time to act.

Will you accept Jesus as your personal Lord and savior?

Sadly, there are people, churches, organizations and, let's face it, certain parts in all of us, that are wimps (have fallen away) or in a state of denial about our sin and the need for a savior. Whether we choose to admit it and seek to change is the important thing.

Remember Romans 3:23

"All have sinned and fall short of the glory of God"

The key word here is **All!**

My preface is that we all need revival in our nutritional approach to what we consume.

As the definition of 'Revival' from *Collins English Dictionary* © *2013* says that it's a reawakening of faith or renewal of commitment to a religion. We need a reawakening, we need to come out of our living death.

Look around you, thousands of people walking through malls, driving in cars, and shopping at stores that are amazingly obese. We are not living in Tonga where obesity is a prized asset. We are in the USA, but this obesity phenomenon is spreading wherever opulence, freedom, and excessive consumerism are prevalent. We, however, don't only need revival in our physical and nutritional side, but in all aspects of our life. Our churches, places of worship, hobbies, financial lives, entertainment choices, emotional vitality; virtually all aspects in our sin filled world that we need to repent and turn from.

I love these verses from Galatians 5:16-24 as it highlights so much about how then we should live by the Spirit of Christ living within us.

"So I say, walk by the Spirit, and you will not gratify the desires of the flesh. For the flesh desires what is contrary to the Spirit, and the Spirit what is contrary to the flesh. They are in conflict with each other, so that you are not to do whatever you want. But if you are led by the Spirit, you are not under the law.

The acts of the flesh are obvious: sexual immorality, impurity and debauchery; idolatry and witchcraft; hatred, discord, jealousy, fits of rage, selfish ambition, dissensions, factions and envy; drunkenness, orgies and the like. I warn you, as I did before, that those who live like this will not inherit the kingdom of God.

But the fruit of the Spirit is love, joy, peace, forbearance, kindness, goodness, faithfulness, gentleness and self-control. Against such things there is no law. Those who belong to Christ Jesus have crucified the flesh with its passions and desires."

The key word is self-control (with God's Word the Bible as your direction) in all aspects of your life.

Let's continue to strive to be in harmony with the Holy Spirit. Any amount of complacent ignorance in your choices or actions, will only lead to a type of idol worship of laziness, pride and excuses. Justified rationalizations that don't get you anywhere. You need to have a desperate desire to change and allow Christ to come in to clean up the mess you've created. Do you now really think it's only 'self-control' or it's allowing God to live within you guiding and controlling your every step?

Are you doing everything you want or letting God direct your path?

_____

_____

_____

What sins stick out to you that you need to turn away from?

_____

_____

_____

Is there any unconfessed sin in your life that you that you'd like to confess?

_____

_____

_____

I consider this book to be a simplified version of getting the philosophy of how you can reconstruct food choices that will honor your body, mind, soul and spirit. Before going any further about the diet, let's jump into the main foundational things to review as the basics.

This diet begins with reconstructing the parts. So please take a moment and answer these questions and pray about the steps you should take from here as your journey begins:

Where in your life do you need Christ Jesus' revival in your life (Spiritually, Emotionally, Physically, Nutritionally, Financially, Relationally, etc.)?

_____

_____

_____

Where do you pray for Christ to help you let go of wrong living?

_____

_____

_____

What is your current reality as you see it?

_____

_____

_____

Verify verses:

Proverbs 14:15 *"A simple man believes anything but a prudent man gives thought to his steps."*

Psalm 139:23 *"Search me, God, and know my heart; test me and know my anxious thoughts."*

What potentially destructive habits are you doing that may be contributing to your current reality?

_____

_____

_____

_____

What do you need to let go and allow God to take control of in your life?

_____

_____

_____

_____

Ask a trusted friend and God to tell you the answer to the question about the habits they see in your life that are contrary to God's will and may be destructive to your health?

_____

_____

_____

_____

Have you accepted Christ as your savior? Have you

repented from all your sins? Have you asked Him to come into your heart and turn away from your wicked ways? Are you seeking His guidance in everything you do? If not, what is holding you back?

_____

_____

_____

_____

_____

_____

_____

What sins did Christ die on the cross for you? Remember, He has forgiven you (if you ask Him and repent).

_____

_____

_____

_____

_____

_____

_____

_____

_____

_____

_____

_____

_____

_____

Please write a prayer that summarizes your love for Christ, your need for Him, your desire to turn from your sinful ways, and your desire to find rest, health, and the fruit of the Spirit (love, joy, peace, patience, forbearance, kindness, goodness, faithfulness, gentleness and self-control) through Him:

_____

_____

_____

_____

_____

_____

_____

_____

_____

_____

_____

2
RECONSTRUCT

"Do you not know that your bodies are temples of the Holy Spirit, who is in you, whom you have received from God? You are not your own; you were bought at a price. Therefore honor God with your bodies."
1 Corinthians 6:19-20

"Give careful thought to the paths for your feet and be steadfast in all your ways."
Proverbs 4:26

It's a very strong statement to say our body is a temple of the Holy Spirit. How then should we take care of our bodies?

And we were bought with a price. What was that price? Jesus dying on the cross for our sins. Is He your savior? Saving you from an eternity in hell....

The above verses were substantial motivators on my journey. Knowing that my body does house the creator of the universe.

WOW. That in itself made me strive to live out the Proverbs 4:26 verse about giving careful thought to my paths and being steadfast in my ways with the ultimate motivator as God.

The veil of the temple was torn. Now the place where God lives is with men, as the Holy Spirit can guide our lives if we give it over to Him. Jesus died on the cross and bore the responsibility for all our sins, so that we could eventually come to fellowship with Him and know Him more.

What an amazing gift for **all** of us!

A sacrifice of greatest price.

Hallelujah!

Praise Him!

Have you invited the Holy Spirit in to help clean, tidy up, and renew your temple? (If not please reread chapter 1)

_____

_____

_____

How are you pondering the path of your feet?

_____

_____

_____

Draw a picture here of how you view your temple:

God can't have sin in his presence since He is perfect. So He made this training ground and testing area for us to see His glory and mighty power, while understanding that our brokenness and sin is only made right by Christ.

This happens only as we turn to Him in everything. Let's start small and look at one thing you can reconstruct in your life.

Looking at the simple equation:
Current Reality = A + B + C + D + E

Applying this equation to my life previously it looked something like this:

Slightly Overweight, Lacking Direction (previous reality)

=

Hard Work @ Everything
+
Trying to Please Others
+
Stressed Out
+
Lacked Control (in eating, emotional responses, goal setting, and follow through)
+
Fearful
+
Trying to Prove My Worth or Value to Others (And getting the praise of the world)
+
Whatever else negative that might be in your life

The new life that you are striving for has a desired outcome and the simple equation is to substitute the items that make your current reality by the outcomes that will get you to your desired Life. (Maybe jot it

down in the cover of your Bible with a date near it.)

Sometimes you may need to effectively deconstruct the parts in order to reconstruct properly.

You've heard it said that professional athletes are working at breaking down their swing, or stance to improve on it. Effective deconstruction is taking a look at your situation and breaking it apart in order for you to allow God to fully work in your life by rebuilding and strengthening you through.

Desired Life = G + O + D

Faithful follower of Christ
(Make my temple a place worthy of Christ to reside)

=

Moving my Faith from my mind to my heart (living it)
(Most important is follow God in my day-to-day
choices…this can come through Bible study,
fellowship, individual prayer, and family prayer.
Nothing compares to the 1-1 intimate time you can
share with Christ through prayer)
+
Following through on tasks God directs me to
(Prayer, prioritization and action, self-control in
choices, working for God and not for the praise of
man)
+
Healthy lifestyle commitment
(Self-control in eating, exercise, and choices, inspired
and motivated by God)

+

Being a better spouse, parent, and friend
Current Reality = A + B + C + D + E

Please write down your current reality (use extra

paper if you'd like too): *these equations are also listed on convenient pages in the back of the book you can print off)

_____

=

_____

+

_____

+

_____

+

_____

Now write the new life that you are striving for with a desired outcome. Substitute the items that make your current reality by the outcomes that will get you to your desired life.

Desired Life = G + O + D

_____

=

_____

+

_____

+

_____

The Christian Revival Diet™ focuses on:

    Ingesting a healthy diet of your burden that God gives you (your ministry, your service and outreach), God's word, God's food, God's direction, God's healthy living, and God's rest in your life.

    Sometimes when you break things down in order to change you have to dismantle it first in order to then rebuild it better, faster, and stronger.

    Isn't it amazing that the same principle applies to weight lifting? In order to build stronger muscles we need to break down muscle fibers to then produce micro tears which in turn are healed stronger than before.

    So is our journey and quest in all areas of our life. To break them down further and simplify in order to strengthen again. I like to say we need to *"deconstruct in order to reconstruct"*.

    There is a Navy Seal mantra that states, *"Fast is slow, and slow is fast."* When you are able to break things down slowly and learn them, your ability to process them faster happens with greater efficiencies. The mastery level is when you are able to do something without thinking. Your unconscious takes over, and you are able to move forward effortlessly. However, if you don't keep pushing your own limits you may end up decreasing your ability and performance.

    A friend of mine, Ryan, a physical fitness trainer and the head of metabolic fitness testing and training at a local gym, explained to me some interesting statistics that spurred me on to develop more of a laser-like focus for training, tracking and focus. His comment was that when you focus on two things at a time, your success rate drops to 20% versus focusing on one thing at a time which raises the chances of successful completion up to greater than 85%. Thanks, Ryan, for your personal mentoring and insight. So when you decide to change the three or four things in your life from the equation, consider it the vision that you are aspiring to work towards, and look at one of the items at a time to better focus your energy and train for that one goal.

This is evident while observing my kids as they are learning sports. They have all been involved in hockey and soccer, and if I as the coach in soccer, have them go out and trap, pass, kick, and turn all at the same time, they get confused and can't do it. The most successful coaches spend the majority of the time focusing on one item at a time, be it a pass, a trap or a quick turn. They integrate these lessons in a series of drills and then return weekly by until the kids are masters of that specific skill.

A coach of mine mentioned that interval training and tapering is very important in achieving improvement in skills. Our goal was to improve our running from eight minutes to under seven minutes for a 10K. We started with a prescribed training method of intervals: sprinting for a mile and then jogging at a slower pace for a mile. The final week before our training we sprinted for three miles and then jogged for one and then sprinted for three again and rested for one. I felt like I was going to vomit at my peak speed for three full miles.

Two weeks later, on a frigid Minnesota February day, we ran it a bit under seven minutes per mile. The frost on my eyelashes was one of the only memories I have after the grueling run. All in all it's amazing what your body, mind, and spirit will adapt to, both positively and negatively. Then six months after this test, I ran a 5k at a personal record, clocking in six minute and ten second per mile. Faster than I had ever run.

When someone is training for a marathon, there is an 18-24 week training period that includes daily running or resting as well as various durations that range from 0 to 18 miles.

Jesus says that the end is near. If we know that our time may come at any day, how are we training for eternity?

_____

_____

_____

What would a typical training schedule look like to get us ready for eternity? What would true solid Biblical training look like if you had to craft a plan for it?

_____

_____

_____

Are you training with the same vigor as the marathoner in light of the coming Day of Judgment, and the fact that the end is near?

_____

_____

_____

Simply ask Jesus to come into your heart and strengthen you in Him. Jesus is the training plan.

Where will you start, what one thing will you focus on first, and why?

_____

_____

_____

_____

Can you break down that into smaller parts to see if there are components that will allow you the chance for greater success?

_____

_____

_____

_____

_____

How would you describe your training plan for eternity?

_____

_____

_____

_____

My goal for the next six months is to keep me refueled with God's spirit by memorizing and being able to recite the entire book of James. Please pray for me, and if you read this after April 21, please pray that I retain the passage and accomplished it.

At this point, let's take a physical and mental check-up to where you are at with your body. This exercise allows you to savor peace and feel any areas of tension or pain in order to gauge them to be able to do something to make it better.

I'd urge you to slow down be observant and prayerful to every breath, sound, sensation for one minute. As you breath in try to count to five and fill your lungs slowly as and then slowly exhale counting to five.

What did you notice? Are you at peace, is your mind calm, can you find a center on Christ?

_____

_____

_____

Start this relaxation practice with small amounts of time, starting with one minute per day until you feel comfortable moving it up to five minutes per day, with the eventual goal of doing it for ten minutes at a time. (Please do not hyperventilate, and if you feel light-headed or dizzy please cease the exercise. Make sure your physician is okay with you doing any of these exercises before beginning.)

You'll be surprised at first at the things that come into your mind- the cravings, thoughts, fears, pains, sensations, memories. Do a body scan, a mind scan, a spiritual scan that basically checking for which areas are relaxed and feel good and which areas could use a bit more health.

I like to choose a memory to meditate too through the process as well. If you want to meditate on a memory verse first like Proverbs 3:5-6 feel free. *"Trust in the Lord with all your heart, lean not on your own understanding, in all your ways acknowledge Him, and he will make your path's straight."*

Depending on the speed of your intonation, try to get into a rhythm with the inhalations and the exhalations.

Many who pray and meditate describe the focus as getting in the now and being fully present in that moment. That is your goal as you start to really know yourself better.

After you get to the ten-minute point of silent prayer, please journal some of these notes:

What sensations do you feel?

_____

_____

_____

What do you need to ask Christ to forgive you for in your life?

_____

_____

_____

Who else could you ask Christ to forgive?

_____

_____

_____

Are there any longings that come to mind that aren't fulfilled? How can you deconstruct them to take action toward your desire and God's will?

_____

_____

_____

Are there any potential destructive habits that are coming to your mind? How will you offer them up to the Lord in order to turn from them and trust Jesus?

_____

_____

_____

_____

_____

_____

_____

What action steps could you take currently that would help you feel God's peace in your life?

_____

_____

_____

_____

_____

Based on your silent time, please take some time to deconstruct and reconstruct some other areas of your life. Add to this list some meaningful goals. List what you will do in order to achieve them:

_____

_____

_____

_____

_____

_____

_____

_____

_____

_____

_____

_____

You must seek and choose personal revival.

A personal revival can only come by allowing Christ to live

in your heart and start from the inside out. Don't worry about a global revival. Begin with yourself.

Imagine you had a new room to decorate however you would like to. Imagine you could choose the color of the walls, the trim, the windows, the shades, the furniture, the flooring, the pictures, the lights, and the ceiling. It was your fresh canvas that you could control. Money was no option and time was no option as well. You could decorate everything to reflect the mood, tone, and vision in your mind. What would you put on the walls? What color would you make it? Who would you invite into the room?

Imagine the room was completely white with nothing on the walls and nothing in it. It'd be easy to start, wouldn't it.

Which do you think is easier do? You come with a bias in every situation. And your bias is based on your.

Truth be told, you can't fully understand the system we live in, because you are completely submersed in it. Your understanding is always inherently biased. But I'd say it's easier to start completely from scratch if you wanted to make it exactly the way you wanted it and didn't have to settle for anything less than your ideal vision of that room.

Some people don't care much about the end result and they never know what they are going to get. Nor do they plan to achieve anything. Well, they do end up achieving something, but it is all happenstance. It may even be something that others prize or value, or may make them some money. But at the end of the day, did they really achieve something significant?

For those of you who start with the end in mind, your plan ends up being a little more efficient. You can assess if you succeeded or failed. If you fail to plan, you plan to fail is a favorite mantra I've heard others say.

If you work without a plan it's much more difficult to determine if you have achieved the success you desire. You end up with results that you may not be desiring.

This goes for raising children, choosing and building your profession, playing a musical instrument, having a healthy family relationship, maintaining positive relationships, playing a sport, healthy eating, or developing a strong faith life. Whatever you choose to do, unintentionally or intentionally, you will end up achieving what you set out to do.

Most of us never have taken the time to really sit down and map out what we are working towards. Sadly and gladly the farther we venture down our path, our responses have all paved a path that is unique to our own.

I say gladly because some, with God's blessing, have chosen wisely and have been rewarded by the peace that transcends all understanding and Christ's love. Some, on the other hand, have chosen poorly and their lives, while full of great learning experiences, have been a serious barrage of striving on a road to nowhere.

After 30 or 40 years all the choices we make will catch up to us, and it's much harder to change our path or venture down another road due to time constraints, responsibilities, and the opportunities that are afforded to us.

I bring up the reminder about eternity because it's truly hard to comprehend an eternal focus in our world and live for Christ in all things. Philippians 1:27 highlights a powerful perspective, *"Whatever happens, conduct yourselves in a manner worthy of the gospel of Christ. Then whether I come and see you or only hear about you in my absence, I will know that you stand firm in the one Spirit, striving together as one for the faith of the gospel."*

Relating this to your life and your current goals what are you working on that needs to be remodeled?

_____

_____

_____

_____

How can you start from scratch or from the beginning? What do you need to throw out (ask for forgiveness and forget)?

_____

_____

_____

_____

Consider your desired life and the efforts you are currently making in that area? Are the goals realistic? Have they been tested, and are you being held accountable in order to insure that you are likely of reaching your goals?

_____

_____

_____

_____

What pictures or inspirational phrases would you put on your walls of your room which would help inspire you as you remodel your life after Christ?

_____

_____

_____

_____

_____

3

REVITALIZE

"Therefore I tell you, do not worry about your life, what you will eat or drink; or about your body, what you will wear. Is not life more than food, and the body more than clothes? Look at the birds of the air; they do not sow or reap or store away in barns, and yet your heavenly Father feeds them. Are you not much more valuable than they? Can any one of you by worrying add a single hour to your life...."

Matthew 6:24-34

Worry....Why worry? Worry chokes the life out of you.

Worry takes you captive and doesn't allow you to move forward with your goals.

The quote above from Matthew is so poignant and you may ask the question, if the body is a temple of God and we should take care of it from 1 Corinthians 6:19-20, why then hear should we not worry about our body. If you didn't achieve the self reflection to the depth that you needed to in chapter 2, you may want to review that chapter again and double your target prayer time in order to channel your worried emotions into a more calm, self-controlled state.

Worry is sin. As it's not having faith and trusting in God's provision and direction. It's one of the most tolerated and vogue sins of our day and gains far too little attention in our lives.

The media adorns it by feeding our fuel for it, the marketplace sells it, and entertainment fulfills it, and we consume all of it without even really being aware of it. We can never have enough worry. If we didn't have worry, what would we think about? The things people worry about most are money, education, their sports teams, stock market, job, job loss, tests, education, status, belonging, making a significant contribution. The insurance industry makes a killing on worry, selling extended warranty plans among other things.

The reality is that accidents happen. Unforeseen things can and will come to fruition.

Another sin is gossip or Godless chatter. These sins that rarely get a good amount of teaching time in our world today from our pulpits.

Now let's get back to worry.

I think the key phrase in the above is about 'worry' and yes, I see that the 1 Corinthians 6:19-20 verse about your body being a temple of God and Matthew 6:24-34 can complement each other very nicely. The essence of taking care of your body is indeed part of not having worry in your life. You will not add one day of your life by worrying. Imagine that God was truly living in you.

My father told me a tragic story about a man whose wife passed away unexpectedly as he was raising four boys. My father asked him how he raised four boys in order to gain some tips as it was challenging enough raising two children (me included). He thought it was a tough scenario that he could glean some information from. My dad loves to tell me the story because it has meant so much to him when situations or issues arise that could cause him worry and strife, and he remembers this man's wisdom and seeks to live it out daily.

The gentleman said that whenever things came up that might begin to cause worry for him, he'd go out walking. Some nights he would walk through the night without sleeping, and the worries would go away.

In applying this to my life I added a couple other things to do to keep in balance.

When worry comes there are three things you can do that will ease the worry.
1) Walk
2) Work
3) Pray

The health benefits of walking are significant and so is work. Prayer surpasses all of them, and we are called in all things to pray. The following verses sum it up quite nicely.

Matthew 21:22 *"And whatever you ask in prayer, you will receive, if you have faith."*

Mark 11:24 *"Therefore I tell you, whatever you ask in prayer, believe that you have received it, and it will be yours."*

John 14:13-14 *"Whatever you ask in my name, this I will do, that the Father may be glorified in the Son. If you ask me anything in my name, I will do it."*

Walking, working and praying has helped me greatly... Sometimes I may stretch and pray, kneel and pray, or just lay down and pray. Walking helps clear the mind and helps refocus on what is most important for right now and chases worry away.

I, too, have spent many nights getting refueled in order to

complete the tasks Christ put in front of me by walking, jogging, or running hills. There is something about exercise that clears the mind and refreshes the spirit to the core by doing these types of activities.

Here are some of my favorite quotes about character:

"The ultimate measure of a man is not where he stands in the moments of comfort, but where he stands at the times of challenge and controversy."

Martin Luther King, Jr.

"Intelligence is not enough. Intelligence plus character – that is the goal of true education."

Martin Luther King, Jr.

"Just do it."

Nike Slogan

1 Thessalonians 5:17 *"Pray continually"*

The word and walk are vital in that as well. So when I don't feel I am in a right place to honor God's will, I will work or walk while praying until I feel like things are getting more tuned to His will. When we got kicked out of the Garden of Eden, we were given a task. We'd have to work, see Genesis 3:16-19

"To the woman He said, 'I will make your pains in childbearing very sever; with painful labor you will give birth to children. Your desire will be for your husband and he will rule over you.' To Adam he said, 'Because you listened to your wife and ate fruit from the tree about which I commanded you, 'you must not eat from it,'

'Cursed is the ground because of you; through painful toil you will eat food from it all the days of your life.
It will produce thorns and thistles for you, and you will eat the plants of the field. By the sweat of your brow you will eat your food until you return to the ground, since from it you were take; for dust you are and to dust you

will return. "'

What has worried you that you could work on or "get your walk on?"

_____

_____

_____

_____

What prayers have you given to Christ regarding your worry?

_____

_____

_____

_____

What would God say about the things you do, the things you eat, the thoughts you think, the friends you associate with, the images that you put into your mind, the prayers you pray? (List some of the items below)

_____

_____

_____

_____

_____

_____

Worry is a sin. Yes, "a sin", just like any other sin. God doesn't like us to live in sin as it means we are not in his presence.

What is keeping you up at night? What do you unnecessarily worry about?

How many hours in a day have you worried about something that never happened?

This next example was a huge wake up call for me.

A friend and mentor of mine, Caryl, was helping me do some remodeling work in my kitchen. We had worked hard for about three hours and then took a break.

While sitting down having a snack, Caryl asked me how things were going with me personally and with my faith walk.

I said that sometimes I worried about how I was going to provide for my family, take care of some of the daily tasks and duties in my life, as well as some other things.

Caryl, without hesitation, said to me point blank "Dave, you don't have Christ in your heart!"

Stunned, I looked at him and kind of choked up, "What?"

He then said, smiling, "If you would have Christ in your heart you would have no fears and no worries. You would have the confidence in every situation through Him that he would provide, guide, and give you the strength you need."

Still stunned, I just looked him.

Caryl continued, "You may have Christ in your mind, or at least the concept of God in your mind and an understanding of His grace extended to you, but you haven't fully let him take over your heart and live in you."

This rocketed me on the search and recognition that I needed to allow Christ to live deeper in my heart and to dwell deeper in my soul. The desire to revitalize our lives is God's hand driving our soul for our insatiable quest we all long for in our lives. Revitalization is the one true need that will complement every aspect of your life insofar as you will be answering God's call that glorifies Him and satisfies your soul.

"Do not conform to the pattern of this world, but be transformed by the renewing of your mind. Then you will be able to rest and approve what God's will is – his good, pleasing and perfect will."
Romans 12:2

Just like we deconstructed and then reconstructed an aspect of your life, we are now going to do that same process-this time using our food choices. A tactical approach relating this to the revitalization in your eating, preparing, and purchasing food is essential as a foundation. We often eat more than three meals a day, often snacking and munching without thinking.

This diet is not about new recipes. It's really a concept that will teach you to think through the process of what you allow into your body and the philosophy of reconstructing healthier choices while being proactive and thoughtful about your diet with the goal of vibrant living for and in Christ.

The fun begins when you can catch the spirit of creativity and your taste buds start to change. You will enjoy eating pure and good food, and you will drop harmful addictions that you didn't even know you had.

Be ready! Depending on each person can take sometimes five to thirty-five days to reprogram your taste buds to life giving foods and determine your cravings. As salt, fat, starch, sugars, and oil are inherent in so many packaged and restaurant prepared foods (dead foods) it is essential for you to recognize that weaning yourself from these items takes time.

You could be addicted to salt, fats, starch, sugars and oils without even knowing it. Food addictions and eating for emotions are probably the greatest lack of self-control our opulent living has given us.

Enjoy the process and keep your eyes on Jesus! Realize that you can't do this on your own. Only with Christ can you go forward to achieve the success that He desires for you.

Your current equation may currently be:
It's important to analyze how you make your current food choices. For many of you it might follow this equation:

Food selection

=

Unthinking
+
Lack of knowledge
+
Eat for taste and cravings
+
Empty calories and pre-packaged convenience (dead foods)
+
Trusting the prepared foods without question
+
(Add other items that describe you or cross out the above)
+
_____
+
_____
+
_____
+
_____

In college, I performed a study of the essentials in a grocery store. The professor had a cross-departmental team that mapped out the store and the nutrient and caloric areas in the grocery store. I was the economist. We also had a geographer and a nutritionist on our team, and it was fascinating how we approached this assignment from various vantage points. The end product was stunning.

The geographer mapped it out, the nutritionist calculated the nutrient rich areas per square foot while I merged the price, nutrient and layout to keep people buying the healthiest items for the best value. What we came up with was simply that over more than 85% of the items in the store are non-essentials (dead foods) that were over-priced, filled with low levels of nutrients, and excessive packaging, salt, oils, preservatives and such. The nice thing about these foods is that they create emotional highs as well are super convenient and have long shelf lives.

The study was never published, and it's been lost to the piles of moving, storage, and years gone by. Nevertheless, even without the empirical data, just motivate yourself to perform a quick qualitative review of what you see at the grocery store.

Ask yourself these questions:

Do I truly need this food?

Will it strengthen me or my walk with Christ?

Will the food choice make me healthier?

Is the food within the budget that I have?

Is the food the best use of my money, time, and resources?

What unintentional costs to my mind, body, spirit, soul, and finances does this food bring to me?

The things we don't need also take our money faster, rob us of nutrients, and leave us craving more, which means more consumption tapping our pocket book and leaving us without mental clarity and focus. It makes us a slave to our cravings yet always unsatisfied.

Not only does it hit our food budget, but the eventual toll we will pay for poor food choices in our bottom line years later (our lost opportunities, mental ineffectiveness, relational strain, finances, our flab, our fatigue, and our health care bills).

When we eat better and healthier, we actually save money and have fewer cravings which in turn saves us more of our resources while keeping our body, mind, and spirit much healthier.

Kids know the right thing to eat until they embrace the wrong thing, and then it's hard for them to change. Imagine what a newborn eats happily until there are given 'counterfeit foods'. They happily scarf down squash, peas, carrots, and other unique mushed stuff.

I performed an experiment with my kids, when they were 1, 5, and 7 years old. It showed some surprising results. With children at these ages the truth is always an impulse away.

Imagine soft rich peanut butter covered in sweet and milk chocolate. I love chocolate peanut butter cups. The only thing that may top those could possibly be freshly made peanut butter chocolate fudge. And should I even pretend to say that my children have any self-control around these morsels? Once anything similar arrives on their plate, it's quickly inhaled and the constant chirping in harmony for "more".

So I started on a path to research and give something to my children that was healthy. Thanks to my father's reengineering (deconstructing and reconstructing) approach to food, here is a foundational Christian Revival Diet™ example.

Applying the formula and philosophy from the Revival Diet would look like this.

Chocolate Peanut Butter Cups

Original Ingredients	Christian Revival Diet™ Substitutions
Sugar	Dash of Unpasteurized Honey, Raw Stevia or no need
Chocolate or powder	Raw 100% cocoa nibs
Cocoa Butter	N/A
Milk Fat	N/A
Soy Lecithin	N/A
Vanilla	N/A
Artificial Flavor	N/A
PGPR	N/A
Emulsifier	N/A
Milk	N/A
Peanuts other	Peanuts, Almonds, or favorite nut(s) or 100% nut butter combination
Dextrose	N/A
Salt	N/A
TBHQ(preservative)	N/A
Similar size	
Calories = 200	Calories = 75
Cost = $1 less	Cost = 0.25 cents or
Questionable nutritional content	Nutrient Packed Revival Food™

Imagine as you deconstruct each food item and question yourself asking would I eat this individual item on its own? So, for example, would you grab a teaspoon of emulsifier and eat it? Or a mix of TBHQ and PGPR and just smile as you are eating?

I looked up what PGPR is and it is a viscous liquid of polyglycerol esters of poly condensed fatty alcohol being used to replace the higher priced cocoa butter since 2006. At this point no long term studies on health have been issued. You can research anything on a label today, and I'd say it's a good thing to do.

I am not a food scientist or nutritionist. I am just a simple man who wants to do the right thing with Biblical, spiritual, nutritional, and economical value. If you want to read more on nutrition I'd recommend search online or go to your library and grab a book each month. Hold it up to the Christian Revival Diet™ Philosophy and you will gain wisdom and clarity.

I'm sure there is a good purpose for many of these random ingredients, but frankly I could care less about Soy Lecithin and I'm sure many people could tell me some of the benefits of it, but the great thing about the Revival Diet™ is basically stay away from what isn't pure, good, and quality, and then you'll achieve a wholesome revival in your eating.

Just start thinking, reflecting and questioning.

Out of the original of thirteen items, we can get a similar but healthier result with three items. The amazing thing is that there are more nutrients in the Revival Diet™ selection than the other, and the actual cost is much less.

Now do the kids like it….?

My kids loved it and now are craving natural goodness, 'living foods' and have even turned away ice cream at some birthday parties.

The true test…. (After you've tried some concoctions on your own) is let a friend or family member do a comparison tasting test. As I run through the third edit of this, I'm going to take a break and make one of these up for me right now again. It tastes so good.

The philosophy of the Christian Revival Diet™ is to again reconstruct by considering all the elements of the food and really dissecting what are the tastes and elements inherent in the original form and what solutions or alternatives might be better on all fronts that can increase nutrition, satisfaction, and good health.

Try this experiment on your loved ones at a family get together. Set out two plates with both items on a plate and ask them to go through all their senses: looking, touching, smelling, and then tasting the items in front of them. With regard to the chocolate peanut butter cups, the most amazing thing with all of my kids, when asked the question, "which tastes more real and more living?" all of them pointed to the homemade version. Then I asked them "which tastes better and makes you crave and want to eat more?" Even our 1 year old pointed to the Christian Revival Diet™ choice **before** his brothers did the same.

I have conducted this test numerous times with my children with various food choices and with similar results. They always enjoy and want the food items that are more in their natural God-created state. The biggest obstacle is that it takes a bit more time to prepare. But the results area always better as food closer to its original state, is healthier. Like an orange is better for your body to digest than orange juice. Each step away from the original state loses nutrients.

Try it on your own with enjoyable experimentation until you get down the knack. I have added various other items to the peanut butter cups (with the goal of 100% raw) to spice this up that they even love better.

You can add:
Adding cinnamon
Lemon or Lime juice (fresh or bottled)
Sesame seeds
Minced up fruit (Kiwi, plum, apple, pineapple, banana, etc.)
Various other nuts
Yogurt

Cherry juice
Coconut flakes

There are even expensive sports nutrition bars that my kids loved so much, and when held up to the Christian Revival Diet™ challenge and taste test, the Revival Diet™ wins.

Let's try another deconstruction/reconstruction example before you begin doing your own. Key lime pie is a favorite summer treat it is simple if freshly made.

Key Lime Pie Original Ingredients	Christian Revival Diet™ Substitutions
Sugar	Dash of Unpasteurized Honey, Raw Stevia or no need
Eggs	N/A
Lime Juice	Fresh Limes or 100%
Lime Juice	
Sour Cream	Yogurt Plain
Condensed Milk	N/A
Butter	N/A
Powdered Sugar	N/A
Graham Cracker Crumbs	Choose one or a combination or individual to your liking: Yellow Sesame Seeds, Ground Golden Flax Seeds, Slivered Almonds
Calories = 450	Calories = 75
Cost = $1.50	Cost = 0.50 cents
Questionable nutritional content	Nutrient Packed Revival Food™

Do you really need the sugar, eggs, sour cream, condensed

milk, butter, powdered sugar, graham cracker crumbs (which have their own list of ingredients that are similar to what isn't needed as well)

To the question of what is more living, and fresher, and healthier, the kids all voted for the Christian Revival Diet's™ nutrient packed food again and again.

Granted, you may think my children were raised on this diet so they are biased towards this. Unfortunately, this is not the case, as we are late arrivers to this new eating habit. Even though my dad showed me some of these tricks more than 7 years ago, I was again late in applying his wisdom. I wanted to experiment to find my own truth through this process. I gleaned much information from hundreds of diet and nutrition books, however, none of the books took this angle to really help us to ponder the path of our choices in a God honoring manner.

Proverbs 4:26 *"Give careful thought to the paths for your feet and be steadfast in all your ways."*

The Revival Diet™ is a springboard to catapult you into the realm of questioning, research, and exploration of the food you eat and serve to your family. It's a bridge between what is current and what is possible. The most amazing thing is that if thousand people read this book, there may indeed be a thousand new recipe applications to one food choice. The experimentation works wonders and is fun.

Here is another interesting experiment for you guys out there.

After mowing the yard in the heat of summer, I might consider enjoying the taste of a refreshing beer. While it tastes good, beer always left me a bit tired after having one, so I didn't really acquire a taste for it. However, a few colleagues and I decided to brew some Witbier that was fruity, spicy and refreshing with awesome body. After making 36 bottles from a kit, and learning the process and the science of making beer, we enjoyed a memorable event as well as very tasty and fresh beer.

So I decided to apply the philosophy to the beer making process. I purchased an ounce of hops @ about the cost of $1 and placed it in a French press. Then I poured hot water over the hops and let it cool down, eventually placing it in the refrigerator to cool. The next day I had an amazing drink with all the vibrancy of a beer without the carbonation, the calories, the alcohol, or the sugars.

The cost as well is almost negligible and after further research at the local beer making supply store, there are hundreds of hop varieties that have with unique tastes. When mixed together they produce some wonderful varied concoctions. The reality is beer is cheap to make! The costs come into account for bottling, shipping, taxes and liability.

Check out the recipe listed below, as a beginner new to this type of recipe, some of these items you might say have an acquired taste.

The joy of these 'beer teas' or 'hop teas' is that I can mix and match. They are super fresh and I can drink them anywhere.

Beer Original Ingredients	Christian Revival Diet™ Substitutions
Malted Barely	Dash of Unpasteurized Honey, Raw Stevia or no need
Yeast	N/A
Sugar	N/A
taste some	Add other spices for could include pepper cardamom, nutmeg, lime/lemon/cherry juice or apple cider vinegar.

If you want carbonation add sparkling mineral water.

Hops	Hops
Preservative	N/A

Similar size	
Calories = 250	Calories =35
Cost = $1	Cost = 0.05 cents
Questionable nutritional content	Nutrient Packed Revival Food™

Isn't' it convenient how strong the alcohol lobby has become? They are one of the only food products that gets an exception from having to put the caloric or nutritional content on their packaging. No nutritional requirements like other packaging. While the manufacturers are forced to put driving vehicles and general health warnings. See what they have to put on certain beverages:

Government warning:
    (1) According to the Surgeon General, women should not drink alcoholic beverages during pregnancy because of the risks of birth defects.
    (2) Consumption of alcoholic beverages impairs your ability to drive a car or operate machinery, and may cause health problems

Imagine what the labeling on alcohol should be:

This drink:

Has one serving but adds no nutritional value
This one serving has 150 calories of processed and fermented sugars
Interferes with your mental clarity
Reduces your body's ability to absorb vitamins and

minerals

May cause a hangover, severe dehydration, vomiting, or death

You may become addicted

May inhibit your body's ability to process fats and produce proteins

May spur hunger and over eating

If consumed excessively may produce other maladies, including:

liver disease, cancer, brain damage, depression, anxiety, diabetes, low blood sugar, night sweats, gout, among other things.

It can lower your body's core temperature and your inhibitions.

It may affect your sleep.

*I have not even listed all of the college antics that this could affect.

I personally, however, enjoy a glass of wine now and then. So I am not saying you should abstain. Life is risk, and many of the above can happen without alcohol. However, I think whatever you should be aware of the consequences.

Let's apply this same analysis to the risks on items with excessive sugar or corn syrup derivatives.

1 serving adds virtually no nutritional value

This one serving has 150 calories of high fructose corn syrup

Interferes with your mental clarity

Reduces your body's ability to absorb vitamins and minerals

You may become addicted

May inhibit your body's ability to process fats and produce proteins

May spur hunger and over-eating

If consumed excessively may produce other maladies, including:

liver disease, cancer, brain damage, depression, anxiety,

diabetes, low blood sugar, night sweats, among other things.

Wow, not much different between the risks of the sugary items or the alcohol. Lest I say, everything should be in balance. With these potential effects, it affords the question, "is the fleeting joy and temporary pleasure even worth the risk?" I do enjoy some rich milk chocolate truffles, spiced corn chips, or some other desserts, but it should be in moderation with my health goals and in balance with my metabolism, and I should know the risks.

No one can eat perfectly. There are herbicides, chemicals, and other items in the air, water, and ground that all can or potentially will have effects on us. We can't avoid them all. But the ones that we do have a choice about us definitely can control and minimize. Like the items that are packaged and sold to us.

The reality is the fact that we started this diet philosophy when our kids were ages 7, 5, and 1 by God's hand of grace he has guided us to help educate them on good choices.

Starting from the empty calorie starved food choices (dead foods) we purchased or prepared in the past, all of my children have enjoyed many packaged candies and have loved them over other items at times. It's a constant struggle.

Let's look at some tortilla chips and how to substitute those:

Spicy Tortilla Chips

Original Ingredients	Christian Revival Diet™ Substitutions
Corn	Corn
Vegetable Oil	N/A
Salt	N/A
Cheddar cheese	Any kind of cheese
Maltodextrin	N/A

Wheat flour	N/A
Whey	N/A
Monosodium glutamate	N/A
Buttermilk solids	N/A
Romano cheese	Above
Whey protein concentrate	N/A
Onion powder	Onions
Partially hydrogenated soybean oil	N/A
Partially hydrogenated cottonseed oil	N/A
Corn flour	N/A
Disodium phosphate	N/A
Lactose	N/A
Natural and artificial flavor	N/A
Dextrose	N/A
Tomato powder	Tomatoes
Spices	Spices or add your fresh hot peppers
Lactic acid	N/A
Artificial color Yellow #6 want to	N/A unless you
	throw in a couple of crayons for color or food coloring (Just/Kidding)
Artificial color Yellow #5	N/A
Artificial color Red #40	N/A
Citric acid	Lemon or Lime
Sugar (I wouldn't)	Honey if needed
Garlic powder	Fresh garlic
Red and green bell pepper powder	Fresh peppers
Sodium caseinate	N/A
Disodium inosinate	N/A
Disodium guanylate	N/A
Nonfat milk solids	N/A
Whey protein isolate	N/A
Corn syrup solids	N/A

Add other spices for

taste some
could include pepper

cardamom, nutmeg,
lime/lemon/cherry
juice or apple
cider vinegar.

Similar size
Calories = 250   Calories =35
Cost = $1.42   Cost = 0.25 cents
Questionable nutritional content   Nutrient   Packed
                                            Revival Food™

By the way, did you know that the artificial colors, Yellow #5 and Red #40, are not even allowed in some European Countries? Scary stuff.

I have chopped up the above vegetables and garlic in a bowl, grabbed a hunk of cabbage (I like the purple cabbage), and then cut a slice of cabbage and dip into the vegetables in order to get the crunch, or I just eat them with a spoon. The best is to first determine what you are going to eat and then eat it. Once you've eaten what you think is a serving, then it's best to wait about twenty or thirty minutes as your stomach takes about that time to signal to the brain that it is satisfied.

If you crave salty or spicy things, I've substituted onions, hot peppers, (many varieties) and other vegetables to give me the crunch along with the flavor. The onion and garlic can give a buttery, spicy, savory and delicious flavor better than any chips in a packaged bag.

Now it's your turn!

What is your favorite packaged food item?

_____

_____

Choose one of your favorite items, and break it down from the original ingredients to the Christian Revival Diet™ Substitutions.

Item
Original Ingredients   **Christian Revival Diet™**
                                  Substitutions

_____

_____

_____

_____

_____

_____

_____

_____

_____

_____

Similar size
Calories =   Calories =
Cost =   Cost =
Questionable nutritional content Nutrient   Packed
                                  Christian   Revival
                                  Food™

It'd be an honor if you emailed me what you did, and how it worked for you. I'll put it on my blog. It's not purely a science, it's more of art form with God's tools as the implements. Maybe that's why they call it the culinary arts? ;)

Consider these simple but timeless truths as gold on your path to fitness, faith, and wellbeing. Losing weight for me was a couple equations that followed this mantra.

Calories in versus calories burned.

If you take in more than you burn you will gain weight, and if you take in less than you burn you will lose weight. Unless you lower your metabolism to an unhealthy level and then it will backfire and your body will hoard calories.

On the calories in side, the greatest help for me was realizing that the nutrient rich foods led my body not to go nutrient malnourished and thus not hoard empty calories and then I was less likely to crave empty calories.

The ratio I considered around this was nutrient density divided by total calories. Out of all the calories you eat, if you eat more nutrient dense foods your body will be happier.

Nutrient Dense / Total Calories Consumed = % of Nutrient Dense Foods

So if my basal metabolic rate* (the base rate your body burns calories just by normal activity) was 1800 calories and I only ate nutrient dense foods for 180 calories and the rest was nutrient dead foods, then my ratio would be 10%. The goal would be to eat 80-90% nutrient rich calories and minimize the nutrient dead foods.

*(You can find out yours from a metabolic fitness trainer at a club or a specialized medical professional with a special evaluation).

In our society today, I consider eating nutrient dead foods to be one of the greatest temptations, epidemics, and challenges facing us today. Especially as so many of the counterfeit or dead foods pack huge calorie counts and have a way of tingling our taste buds. So, remember to eat more nutrient dense foods than nutrient dead foods.

Healthy living =
sleep + prayer + activity (service, fellowship, work, exercise) + water + oxygen – distractions – poor nutrition – negative habits

When it comes to weight loss and weight maintenance the best and most helpful things that guided me along the path are listed below.

*Special note before beginning an exercise or nutritional program, check with your physician, medical provider, and or personal trainer to develop a plan that is right for you. Don't take this as specific advice. Please consult them before starting any physical program. This is only a testimony about what it did to help me and may not apply to everyone else. So if these don't fit you, I encourage you to come up with your own top 10 that help you get the success you desire.

1.   Exercise : Minimum 20 minutes of cardio per day

I used to work out when I felt like it. Before having children it was typically either in the morning, over lunch hour, or in the evening. The evening was nice as it was like a double date for my wife and me. This was fine without children in our lives! However, as they graced our family I wanted to spend more of their waking hours with them. I would work out when I felt like it. With the demands of my day it ended up often being late at night between 9 p.m. and 1 a.m. when the duties were done and the kids were sleeping.

One day I had enough and said that I would do the number of pushups per year as every year I'd been alive. I also planned to do sit ups every morning before work and at least 20 minutes of cardio. So I had to leave the house earlier, between 4:30 and 5:30 a.m. to get my workout in. Then I joined the fitness club, and it became easier.

Now I'm often at the fitness club 1-2 hours of 5-6 days per week. There I do my Bible study and quiet time there as well, and all the pre work grooming and such.

The health benefits have been amazing, and the cost of the club probably earns me money instead of costs. I feel healthier, I'm more focused and while it costs $40/month after the insurance reimbursement, our family natural gas bill has been reduced by $30/month now that I shower at the YMCA every morning. So the net $$ cost is about $10/month and I feel like a $1,000,000, inflation adjusted!

2. Sleep : minimum 6-8 hours per night

I am the type of person who doesn't like to sleep. It takes time away from other things that I need to complete and want to do. However, as my friend the physical trainer said "80% of your metabolic functions happen when you sleep". That made me remember that sleep is a very important component of health as it's about recovery, rebuilding, refreshing and ultimately about revival.

Even Jesus, after preaching to the masses, retreated to the mountains to pray and get rest. See Matthew 14:23

On the boat while the waves were crashing, Jesus was sleeping. See Mark 4:38

In the garden before He was going to die for our sins, he was resting. See Mark 14:32-42

On the seventh day even God rested. Wow, if God and Jesus even rest how much more important is it for us. See Genesis 2:2-3

It's one of God's Ten Commandments too! Those Ten Commandments are very important to live by and seek to follow. We hold them up to our lives to convict us of our need for a Savior and the recognition of our sin.

Exodus 20:8-11
"Remember the Sabbath day by keeping it holy. Six days you shall labor and do all your work, but *the seventh day is a Sabbath*

to the LORD your God. On it you shall not do any work, neither you, nor your son or daughter, nor your male or female servant, nor your animals, nor any foreigner residing in your towns. For in six days the LORD made the heavens and the earth, the sea, and all that is in them, but he rested on the seventh day. Therefore the LORD blessed the Sabbath day and made it holy."

I am a poor example on the sleep side, but during the weight loss contest I would discipline myself to get at least 6 hours of sleep each night.

A normal healthy sleep routine is six to eight hours and for each of you it's important to find that balance. Too much sleep can be a bad thing, too, for those of you who are in the camp, I'm not sure I can identify with you. As I think in almost 43 years of living, I've rarely slept in past 8 a.m. on a Saturday or Sunday. So just set your alarm clock a bit earlier and get moving.

For those of you like me who find it hard to get to sleep early, set up a routine to follow that can help you. Brush your teeth early, set your alarm clock as a reminder that will tell you what time you should go to sleep. Then lay down and go to sleep. If you aren't able to, do something that will help you sleep. I've found reading some scientific textbooks or performing deep sleep yoga routines helps considerably. The textbooks are from the past, but the yoga is from the internet I just did a search on Youtube.com and found a night time yoga routine. It's awesome and at this time it is free.

My friend who is a rehabilitation physiologist also mentioned to me that your body needs to repair itself electrically, so any impingements in your neurons can start atrophy in parts of your body as well. Thanks Captain Rob! So it's important that sleep is full, relaxed, and refreshing.

3. Eating a bigger breakfast (including protein for

healthy muscle rebuilding) after my work out and having portion control throughout the day. (Eating smaller portions of the healthy food)

Before starting this diet and revival lifestyle, I used to skip breakfast and sometimes even lunch and work through the day without even taking breaks to stretch. It was an extremely poor health habit and led to apathy, negativity, weight gain, and lethargy.

The side effects of skipping breakfast slow your metabolism down and then when you gorge later because you are so hungry. The body has been put into fear more where cortisol and a "fight or flight" state and you start storing extra calories as your body prepares for you to skip another meal.

What was happening to me physically was that I was starving myself, and then my body would binge to fill the void. The best scenario, I found, is to get the metabolism working right after waking up or right after working out in the morning.

Having a good balance of vegetables, proteins, and carbs first thing signals to your body that there's no need to hoard. You are giving the body and all the organs what they needs. Therefore, the body feels there is no need to store fat!

4. Not eating or snacking after dinner (post 8 pm)

Another thing easier said than done.

Your metabolic functioning occurs best when on an empty stomach. As well, the nights I don't consume food after about 8 pm, I sleep better, feel better when I wake up, and everything else functions better. The other challenge is that once I taste something sweet or salty before bed, I end up eating the opposite like a tennis game. Back and forth, back and forth. Some peanuts, some ice cream, some yogurt, some pretzels until I'm full. Best to close the kitchen and the mouth to food after 8 p.m. Let your body rest to refresh and fully metabolize.

That's why it's good after you eat to tell yourself the kitchen is closed. Brush your teeth, and if you crave something, enjoy a cool glass of water. Speaking of that.....

5. Drinking enough water

Your body is mostly composed of water. Without it you will die rapidly. It lubricates, saturates, transports, and urinates waste products out. Diuretics like coffee, tea, alcohol, are things that dry you out and slow you down.

So make sure you drink enough water and avoid the other items.

6. Eating vegetables as one of the core elements of the food group.

Your mom tells you that you should eat them. Isn't that enough?

7. Eating protein (in the form of legumes, meat, nuts, fish, eggs, etc.)

Protein helps build and repair your cells but if you eat too much it can turn to fat. But most people don't get enough of the good protein. So eat healthy protein such as the above.

8. Weighing myself every morning

By tracking my weight every day, it helps to insure the goal that I am striving for. If I go too much astray, I can quickly get back on track. It is helpful to determine if I need to make more of an adjustment to achieve the goal healthfully. Take it with a grain of salt, your weight can fluctuate plus or minus five pounds per day, depending on your intake of various items (water, starches, sugars, meat, and other items) so don't get frustrated!

Look at a longer term trend. However make sure to track it daily so you can see a trend and start to get to know the fluctuations as well as with your food intake for a while, and it's amazing how you learn more about how your body processes food.

9. **Limiting or completely abstaining from processed wheat, sugars (all), processed foods, and starches for a period of time.**

Many of these refined sugars, wheat, processed foods, and starches have very limited nutrition so don't eat things that might not give you the nutrient content that you desire. Even if it's for a time, I recommend abstaining from some of the items to see how much better you feel.

10. **Praying daily and memorizing scripture with a goal of applying it to your life.**

Prayer changes things, and relying on God's word can give you the strength to handle life's challenges and proceed with strength. The key is in the application. Finding God's will to the situations that come to you and realizing what God wants you to do to work through, overcome, or grow from the situation, will help.

I had to inspect what I expected.

I expected success and I wanted to achieve my goal, however, in light of the accomplishments, I was striving for accountability and when I told myself that failure was not an option, that is when things started to change, and I looked to Jesus for comfort through the trials. I needed to become accountable.

Which meant I tracked my weight daily, my food and daily. The first 21 days were the toughest as my cravings and taste buds were changing. That was also the hardest as my old sugar, salt, and fat cravings (addictions) were creating tough temptations at the grocery stores, and as I drove by every fast food restaurant.

In tracking I simply used these items:

AM Weight	Exercise Time	Calories Taken In	PM Weight

I also gave myself a grace day once (and sometimes twice) per week to eat whatever I wanted. Which was met with old favorites like cookies, pie, ice cream and such sweet things that were not a rarity in my old world of eating. These grace days always though led to more temptations and slips.

The first 30 days I lost about 15 pounds, the second 30 days it was about another 15 pounds, and more importantly than the mass or the actual weight was the healthy feeling I was experiencing. I felt more attune to what God had for me to do in my life, as well all many of the mid-life aches and pains were gone. Praise God!

My physical fitness trainer, who runs the metabolic testing program at a local club, mentioned to me that many folks have a gluten allergy which causes ligaments to swell. As I nourished my body with better nutrients, limited the gluten and reduced the weight, my body was working so much better and feeling so good. I even went running for about ten miles and didn't have any of my normal joint aches.

It felt like I was 21 years old again, ½ of my age.

Isn't that so often the case, rather than wait for the item that is better and defer our gratification, we will jump to the item with immediate satisfaction.

Remember Proverbs 27:7

"He who is full loathes honey, but to the hungry, even what is bitter tastes sweet."

As I write this at 6:12 a.m. on a Sunday, I have a mammoth bowl of alfalfa, clover, and fenugreek sprouts sitting next to me. As I bite a mouthful, the spicy water from each sprout has a sweet calming taste. Next to me is a white chocolate chip peanut butter oat bar about a 1 inch by 1 inch size. The sprouts have about 1/10th the calories and are at least 4 inches by 6 inches wide.

As I taste a nibble of the white chocolate.... bar, it's like explosions of happiness going into my mind saying more... more... more. And I then proceed to eat more until that bar, the little 1 inch square is gone, but my mind is saying more and more. No satisfaction. Did I only eat for taste? Why does my mind send the pleasure signals so rapidly to my mind?

I brought the bar home from a pot luck from the afternoon before. The interesting thing is that there were three pre-teenage girls, unsupervised, next to me in line at the potluck. They were ravaging and cleaning out the pan full of the chocolate bars. Their ages, I guessed, ranged from 10 to 12. I happily commented, "Those taste so good". One responded, "Once you eat one, you just can't stop!" They were smiling as they were stuffing their faces.

When you eat for taste you will crave more and your desires will almost never be met. But it's so difficult for any choice. At that pot luck there were 12 different chilies to taste (it was a chili cook off) at least twelve different bags of chips and about seven pans of bars, cookies or desserts. Really, what hope did the children have? What choice were they going to spend their choices to eat? How many were going to have seconds of the spicy chili with onions, cheese, and sour cream? In comparison to the sweet buffet of desserts? By the way, this was a devout group of Christians at a fellowship.

My father even said once to me, that most women out of love through diet cook to kill their husbands. The buffet line is a telling sign. Compared to 190 years ago we are now consuming a lot more sugar. A study found on Business Insider done by Stephan Guyenet and Jeremy Landen found that we *'in 1822, the average American ate the amount of sugar found in one of today's 12-ounce sodas every 5 days. Now, we eat that much every 7 hours.'* Which means a 15-18 fold increase in the amount of sugar consumed. And it is growing every day. You find concession stands children's baseball games, vending machines in school, church lobbies filled with cafes, and people trying to give candy and cookies at every event.

After the smoke clears from this assault on our bodies. What remains is increased diseases starting now with children at younger ages: obesity, diabetes, ADHD, lack of sleep, other diseases not even yet identified as caused by this unprecedented overuse on our kidneys, liver, spleen and insulin production. With what effects this has on our body, we may wake up one day and ban sugar as an illegal drug.

I would even say that whoever cooks for their family or shops for them and are ignorantly unaware at what they are doing help to slowly kill their kids and themselves. The statistics show that a very large percentage of children today will end up with type 2 diabetes is direct effect of eating for the tastes.

Are there any things that you tell yourself you can't live without? Are there any impulses or cravings that you know you shouldn't take part in that you do?

_____

_____

_____

_____

Could you go one day without that food, that thing, that item?

_____

_____

_____

_____

If you had to rate your nutritional consumption on a scale of 1 to 10, 10 being nutrient packed and 1 being junk food junkie, which would you rate it today?

_____

_____

Self-denial, deferring gratification, and living simply can be hard concepts in practice for everyone. Especially in an overly packaged society where most everything is made for shelf life and taste. After the first 21+ days on the new diet, trust me your taste buds will change, and you will actually start to crave broccoli for a snack, or some savory kale, or that big bowl of sprouts.

Fasting is an important part of growing in self-control. James MacDonald, pastor of Walk in the Word Ministries and Harvest Church, had a great sermon, called *"The Discipline of Fasting"* archived on Oneplace.com where he highlighted that nothing should control you but Christ. And if anything does in fact control you, it may not allow your relationship to Christ grow as much as it could.

When is the last time you have deferred gratification in your eating? (By fasting or abstaining from a certain food?)

_____

_____

_____

_____

When is the last time you have deferred gratification in some other area of your life? (By fasting from entertainment or a hobby or something)

———————————————————————————————

———————————————————————————————

———————————————————————————————

———————————————————————————————

How did you feel after you abstained from that area?

———————————————————————————————

———————————————————————————————

———————————————————————————————

With the sprouts, although my mind doesn't say more...more...more, I know that my stomach says "thank you" and three to four hours later, my body will have the energy and vigor to say a loud and clear "thank you".

It's calming and refreshing.

What food today do you not like that you should? And vice versa?

———————————————————————————————

———————————————————————————————

———————————————————————————————

———————————————————————————————

Again, please do not to be too extreme. I did eat the one inch white choco-peanut butter thing today, and had the urge to eat as much that would fit on a plate would linger, had it been available. But I also ate the sprouts and I limited myself when my body said go for the next chocolate bar.

Everything in moderation and balance is also something my father frequently commented and reinforced to me as a child. The challenge becomes, isn't it funny how we all have our own definitions of moderation? We continually shift that moderation depending on the group we are with, the emotions we are feeling, and the things that we encounter, the tasks at hand, and the situation and what we want. So is it true balance or a societal balance that we want?

Our sense of stability regarding the conflict between nutrients and junk food is in the magnitude of a cosmic battle between good and evil. As eating is one of the foundational aspects of our survival, we tend to not consider things we eat as either good or evil just more of what have you done for my taste buds lately? Now it's time to revitalize.

The reality is that be it what goes in your mouth, eyes, and ears it all goes into building the person you are, and the consequences are real for all of us.

Some even have the arrogance to say *"live for today as tomorrow you will die, why not enjoy the moment and have no regrets"*. I have personally lived that way in many areas of my life and at many times. I know the regrets from this style of living.

Jesus says in Matthew 6:21-24 some amazing words:

"For where your treasure is, there your heart will be also. The eye is the lamp of the body. If your eyes are healthy, your whole body will be full of light. But if your eyes are unhealthy, your whole body will be full of darkness. If then the light within you is darkness, how great is that darkness!

No one can serve two masters. Either you will hate the one and love the other, or you will be devoted to the one and despise the other. You cannot serve both God and money."

And in Psalm 24:4-5 is declares:

"The one who has clean hands and a pure heart, who does not trust in

an idol or swear by a false god. They will receive blessing from the Lord and vindication from God their Savior."

But after eating the bar, I must admit I don't fell as good as I think I could have. For example, what we give up with those 2-4 seconds of pleasure gulping down that sugar, is a sustained feeling of energy and well-being. However for me I regret it less eating it at 6:32 a.m. before my workout than eating it at 8:45 p.m., and then not be able to stop until three or four of the bars are ingested.

Your personal path may be a bit different, your challenges may be a bit different. You may have different goals, genetics, cravings, etc. It is ok to be patient with yourself, ask for forgiveness, and to learn what is the best for your body, soul, and mind. You will learn how the Holy Spirit will use you for His glory in Christ's balance for you.

Special note: I did purchase a $5 scale from the discount department store to weigh items to see what the approximate calorie and weight equivalents are. Truthfully, I probably used three times to get a sense for serving sizes and the weight and calorie density of things. After that I just ball parked the weight and serving size. I also tracked everything I ate for the first three months with daily morning and evening weigh in on my own scale.

There are also smartphone applications that can journal these things easily. My parents did the same thing but with a book on foods in a prayer and diet journal. Their outcomes were wonderfully successful, and frankly their inspiration helped lead me down this path.

Imagine if your mind, body, and soul had their own conversations with each other? What would each area ask or say to each other?

The mind is easy to think about, but it's extremely difficult for us to fully perceive our state of being and what others think of us or see us as. It's difficult for us to fully realize our strengths and weaknesses. But we can speak to our mind and have an immediate change.

Our body takes more time to build up strength, rebuild, and become stronger. We can't just tell or think our body to be healthier, we need to take care of it. While it does more things than we can even fully comprehend. It reminds us how much of what our mind leads us to our state of physical shape.

Our soul, on the other hand, is the most important! It means so much to God to keep everything in check that Moses wrote it in the Old Testament.

In Deuteronomy 6:5 *"Love the Lord your God with all your heart and with all your soul and with all your strength."*

As well, Jesus spoke the same quote when asked what the greatest commandment, he replied, *"Love the Lord your God with all your heart and with all your soul and with all your mind".*

So are you loving God with your heart, your soul, and your mind? How and where can you love Him more in your life?

_____

_____

_____

_____

This is your diet and God can lead you, if you strive and hunger and thirst for His righteousness. One step at a time.

Trust Him!

4

RETRAIN

**"If the people let government decide
what foods they eat and what medicines they take,
their bodies will soon be in as sorry a state
as are the souls of those who live under tyranny."
Thomas Jefferson**

What would make Thomas Jefferson write such a quote? Is it the fact that he understood that government uncontrolled would restrict freedoms and in essence extend its control with too great a force to otherwise become tyrannical or over controlling?

I can't believe there could be such a state or situation when someone else would in essence control you. However, any cursory look at history shows ample examples of tyranny and oppressive government imposed controls around the world.

The worst and most dangerous controls are subtle, unconscious collections of our own acceptance, tolerance, and our deafening silence by not challenging, questioning, or standing firm in our convictions or God's direction for your life.

Let me propose here that the philosophy of our consumption of not only food is in a dangerous state, but also other areas of what we consume: our information, our entertainment, our ideologies, our guiding tenants, our politics, and our unconscious awareness. And you thought this was just another diet book, no my friend, this book indeed has the goal of revival questioning our fundamental foundations of our freedoms and why we do what we do. (Or what we don't do, too)

We are living in a fallen world, where Satan, the father of lies, is wielding his power.

I stand firm in saying that responsible freedom of choices are indeed the basis for the best society we can ever hope to live in this side of heaven. God gave us freedom to choose to sin, or choose Him.

It's your choice.

However, freedom without control is anarchy; control without freedoms is tyranny. So where should we find balance and our peace? In Christ. You may ask, how do we live the Christian life? Put simply Christ is the Christian life....John 14:6 *Jesus answered, "I am the way and the truth and the life. No one comes to the Father except through me."*

So when you are thinking of all the choices you make and the things that you do or think you should do (Bible studies, church, music, work, fellowship, work, friends, social, TV, hobbies, computer use, etc.)

What is really the most important?

_____

_____

_____

Christ is the most important.

So how are you living the Christian life today? How is your relationship with Christ?

_____

_____

_____

_____

_____

_____

What does God want you to start doing today?

_____

_____

_____

_____

What does he want you to stop doing?

_____

_____

_____

_____

"Do not conform to the pattern of this world, but be transformed by the renewing of your mind. Then you will be able to test and approve what God's will is – His good, pleasing and perfect will."
Romans 12:2

Jesus loves us and wants us to come to Him no matter how many times we have strayed and failed. In so many ways the United States has fulfilled this mission. Relating it to food choices, yes, if someone wants to eat horrible things by choice, then let them choose and live with the consequences. And yes the consequences can be dyer when you make that same poor choices for many years. However, our nation's wealth has given a buffer to extend grace to those in this situation. Our nation has safety measures (such as medications, surgeries, dialysis, insulin, top quality social services and psychological care and other medical and technological breakthroughs) to help those who make bad choices better. Nevertheless, the costs do affect all of us and our loved ones and will for generations to come.

Think about this....

Consider these numbers
1
2
4
8
16
32
64
128
256
512
1024
2048

What is the pattern here?

Simply put this is a pattern for doubling each previous number.

If you go back three generations from me that would be my parents, my grandparents, and great grandparents. That would be 8 great grandparents if they were living that would be related to me. So if you go back to great, great, great, great, great, great, great, great, great-grandparents, unless we lived in the save village our whole life and did some dangerous inbreeding, we'd have 2048 great times 9 grandparents.

Now if the average generation is 20-25 years guess going back two-thousand to Jesus' time how many relatives we would have if we had 78 times great grandparents?

Now consider this, if God will punish generational sin to the third or fourth generation, and extend grace and forgiveness to all who believe, imagine the importance of everything that you do and how it affects your children's children.

"You shall not bow down to them or worship them; for I, the Lord your God, am a jealous God, punishing the children for the sin of the parents to the third and fourth generation of those who hate me, but showing love to a thousand generations of those who love me and keep my commandments." Exodus 20: 5-6

It is highlighted in Exodus 34:7 and Numbers 14:18 as well as Deuteronomy 5:9.

For generations....

Our time here is relatively short, and our influence on the world around us very small.

A man once said that you will be missed as long as the impression of your hand remains in a bucket of water as you pull it out. The world fills in around you rapidly.

This convicted me in my own self-centered vantage point to the world and lives around me. I can name my parents, grandparents, a few of my great grandparents and only a couple of my great, great-grandparents. I'm sure this will change going forward when you consider that technology allows genealogy to be traced more easily.

But the reality is that the reliance on parents and grandparents to imprint meaningful stories and lessons from those that came before them is paramount to help children and your children's children from avoiding the mistakes of previous generations.

As a child my life consisted so much of peer dependency, Hollywood's entertainment, sports or games. At some times those became the most important social interactions. Much more than the roots of the family.

We are all part of a larger group of people searching for meaning or shared meaning default to potentially erase their histories, cultural aspects and in so many cases their faith for the immediate. It's easy to be open to anything new, when you have no heritage or history. Maybe that is why history repeats itself on the macro level as well as on the individual level. We repeat the same mistakes individually even perhaps more often.

So again at 78 times great grandparents how many would that actually be? Write your guess

---

I know when you see the number it will seem flawed. As the first question that I had when I saw it was that there was not even that many people ever alive!

Upon further reflection that is indeed true, but that is because of generational overlap and intermarrying relatives third or fourth cousins sharing same great-grandparents.

I'm not saying to go back and become an enclosed society. There are many benefits of being a global society and being able to travel and be connected to many people. Imagine my great-great grandfather, Johannes Engler came from Switzerland in about 1868 following the footsteps of his younger brother David Engler who traveled from Switzerland about 4-5 years earlier.

The trip from Switzerland might have been to Holland by train or by horse, or by foot. It is estimated that the ships journey from Switzerland would have taken at least 10-14 days just to leave a port on the European continent and arrive in Nova Scotia. Johannes took the risk even though his Brother David's ship sunk off the coast before David ever arrived on the North American continent.

Johannes then took some means of transportation to

southern Wisconsin, where he settled on a small farm and meagerly survived working the land, milking the cows, and enjoying time with his family.

As a youth I dreaded visiting dusty court houses and cemeteries to trace the marriages and see gravestones. But before the internet, this was the only way my father's mission to trace the family roots. It has been a blessing for me as 18 years after my father traced our roots, my wife and I were married in the church of my great-great grandfather in Sevelen, Switzerland.

The reason I am highlighting this is that our roots are important, and we can learn a lot from them. My great-great grandmother had roots in Norway. My parents were able to visit that farm that had only been accessible across a frigid fjord by an oar boat. I haven't yet visited there, but my prayers are that someday my current family could spend more time in there to get a flavor for life of my ancestors.

Nevertheless, if people never had shared great or great grandparents the number listed below, as happens with pedigree collapse.

Here is the number without that collapse.

1,200,000,000,000,000,000,000,000

That's 1.2 Septillion. 12 with 23 zeros, which is amazing to think of how many people have connected in order to make you and lead you to this place in history. We truly stand on the shoulders of giants as Isaac Newton mentioned.

I wish I knew the stories of their lifestyles, their history, migrations, pains, and toils. But mostly I wish I could thank them for living well.

We have all been given privileges and rights and we must have honor and duty to fulfill these privileges and rights. Freedom without self-control or boundaries is anarchy.

Control without freedoms is tyranny. Finding the balance is the challenge.

Our unfortunate reality, however, is that so many people in our country trust without verifying. They (we) buy without considering. They (we) eat without thinking. We (they) talk without reflecting. They (we) watch and accept what they see without questioning.

A strong Christian friend of mine loves to memorize Bible verses. He reminds me on the value of Biblical instruction and teaching.

These verses are the two that he likes to remind me of often, and I believe the Bible gives us a basis for retraining the programming that has already been socialized into our modern day existence with the goal of resetting our path to God's will – His perfect and pleasing will.

Let's start with these two verses:

2 Timothy 3:16 *"All scripture is God-breathed and is useful for teaching, rebuking, correcting and training in righteousness"*

What does this mean to you?
How can you apply this to your life?

_____

_____

_____

2 Timothy 4:2 *"Preach the word; be prepared in season and out of season; correct, rebuke and encourage = with great patience and careful instruction"*

What does this mean to you?
How can you apply this to your life?

_____

_____

A friend of mine, Jack, also pointed out to me that it is helpful to focus on this verse to help steer our direction and path. Looking with expectation and obedience to God for what he has planned for us. By studying and reviewing God's words, we strengthen our step to better self-control and questioning and acceptance.

"Whatever is true,
whatever is noble,
whatever is right,
whatever is pure,
whatever is lovely,
whatever is admirable
– if anything is excellent or praiseworthy –
think about such things."

Philippians 4:8

Let's read the opposite side of this verse to understand potential areas we may fall victim:

"Whatever is false, negative or counterfeit,
whatever is lowly or shameful,
whatever is wrong or inappropriate,
whatever is not genuine or polluted,
whatever is hateful and fearful,
whatever is unworthy and despicable
– if anything is inferior or dishonorable –
Act upon such things without foresight."

Living in your sinful nature

My rendition (with some additions) of this verse may sound a bit extreme or harsh, but sometimes deconstructing or looking at the inverse or opposite can help us realize the true reflection of the choice we make and make our choices more intentional.

Seeing this inverse actually makes the magnitude of God's grace and the purity of His love even more awe inspiring. I like to consider this inverse as a 'deconstruction'. It can be applied in so many areas such as food, politics, opinions, nutrition, faith, sciences, information technology, economics, and so on.

What stands out to you on some of the areas of the differences of between the Philippians verse and the inverse?

_____

_____

_____

_____

Colossians 3:2-4 highlights another timeless truth to consider:

"Set your minds on things above, not on earthly things. For you died, and your life is now hidden with Christ in God. When Christ, who is your life, appears, then you also will appear with Him in glory."

Which verse above tends to display your mindset?
God's word or the inverse?

_____

_____

_____

Where would you like to grow along these lines?

_____

_____

_____

I use the term, "counterfeit action" to describe any thought, word, deed that pulls us into our sinful state of being.

Yes, I believe a thought is an action. The biomechanics and chemical reactions that occur in your mind has proven this. However as a non-scientist, let's try this experiment together.

Imagine tasting a lemon in your mouth......

What happens to your saliva? What happens to your mouth?

Now what about imagining tasting a sweet and tart cherry?

What do you feel around your lips, cheek, and gums?

For me, I feel the sensations and saliva build up almost as if the food is in my mouth. While it's a non-caloric nerve and taste bud reaction, I personally can taste the sour flavor in my mouth.

Another quote from Jesus that summarizes this point well is in Matthew 5:28-28; *"You have heard that it was said, "You shall not commit adultery. But I tell you that anyone who looks at a woman lustfully has already committed adultery with her in his heart."*

There are those who try to argue that being tempted isn't a sin, I completely disagree with this. Once you acknowledge something is a sin, you've indeed sinned as your thought life has termed it as bad, and you have consciously identified it as such. So beware and be careful, please.

When Jesus says this about your thought life, it paints the importance of making each thought pure and righteous. Just because someone else may not know what you are thinking, doesn't mean that God isn't judging that thought or that intention.

Gandhi's quote about beliefs is powerful. Holding this up to God's standard and desire for us, please consider:

"Your beliefs become your thoughts,
Your thoughts become your words,
Your words become your actions,
Your actions become your habits,
Your habits become your values,
Your values become your destiny."

Where are or have your thoughts are become your destiny?

_____

_____

_____

_____

_____

What are you thinking about today that could be changed?

_____

_____

_____

_____

_____

When hiking a volcano one autumn, named Mt. Chokai in Northwestern Japan, I witnessed some of the most beautiful contrasting colors as the reds, greens, browns, silvers, blues, and whites all swirled up and down the majestic contours of the mountain on my hike. Every view I looked was a complete wow moment. Like a photo shoot for the world's most colorful and scenic wild mountain environments.

My Japanese guide, told me the term "Chowa", which means a contrast with harmony. When there is a stark contrast we can see the separation much better. Thus making an inverse helps us see the distinctions and separation more clearly. The deeper the contrast the greater it separates.

Would you be able to commit to one week not saying anything without truly considering the Biblical filter and Christ's blessing on what you are about to say?

If a week sounds too challenging break it down and try perhaps a day, an hour or even a minute to start. If yes add the date and time you will try to begin and what happened through the process.

_____

_____

Would you be able to commit to one week (or a shorter duration) not eating a specific food, or drink that might not be healthy for you? If yes, add the date and jot down what happened?

_____

_____

My prayer around this action would read like this:

"With God's help and strength,
  Whatever is true, I will aim to do!
  whatever is noble, allow my eyes to behold,
    whatever is right, let me strive with might,
      whatever is pure, let me love to do,
        whatever is lovely, God bless my steps,
      whatever is admirable, let my strength encumber,
if anything is excellent or praiseworthy – let me not stray
  think about such things and do without delay."

Philippians 4:8
+ after the comma's my prayer

Here is an example of retraining your mind in line with the Philippians verse above, moving from the worldly negative flow of thoughts to the true, noble, right, pure, lovely, admirable and praiseworthy areas of your life.

To really focus on retraining our minds deconstruct a

previous conversation or previous thought that you may have had in a certain circumstance and then reconstruct the situation with the application of Philippians 4:8.

Here is an example I have thought relating to my job performance and how I'm valued by my manager or supervisor over the years.

Some of my old thoughts, "counterfeits" and negative self-talk:

They don't appreciate my hard work
I don't do as well as someone else
I want to get the most out of it whatever I can
I want to help others
I don't have much to offer
They don't really appreciate me
I'm not doing as well as I could
My contributions aren't very valued
I don't feel appreciated for what I do
I'd like more recognitions, awards, and praise in my work
I'm impatient with getting what I feel I want
I'll never get to fulfill my potential
I'll never achieve the level of success I deserve
They won't achieve the standards that we need to hit
I don't have boundaries
My employer doesn't really need me at the workplace

Add some of your counterfeit thoughts below (and circle those above that apply to your life as well):

_____

_____

_____

_____

Another equation that I equally enjoy is

Success = Potential (the gifts God has given you) – Distractions or the Interference

Success must, in this scenario, mean the reality of comprehending God's path for your life and living and striving for Him and His direction with a hunger and thirst that are only quenched through Him.

Thus the focus on positive self-talk is vital. But it only holds merit when doing our best to hold it through God's lenses on what He truly wants us to do in even the simplest situation.

Positive and new self-talk:

God has a plan for me
I can handle all things through Christ who gives me strength
I work with all my strength to the Lord
I seek praise from God for my contributions
I learn from others and do the best I can
I trust my contributions will be valued in God's timing
What little I have, I will give to help support the cause for Christ
I want to do God's will daily in my life
I will wait on recognition and praises in my work in God's timing
I have hope and faith the following God's direction will prevail
I can do it with the one who gives me all things
My contributions will help the team
We can do this
I can set proper priorities
I can wait for deferred gratification
I have strong will power
I am not afraid, I have faith in light of the challenges

Add some of your positive self-talk here:

_____

_____

_____

_____

_____

_____

_____

Thoughts are so powerful and once they become set into us, it is a challenge to break free from them. A quote from John Maynard Keyne's Book called *"The General Theory of Employment, Interest and Money, Preface, p. viii (1936)*, John highlights:

"The constant struggle of escape from habitual modes of thought and expression, the problem lies not in the absence of new ideas, but breaking free from the old ones, which ramify, for those brought up as most of us have been, into every corner of our minds."

Keynes' made his point so effortlessly and leaves us compelled to continue to question, reflect, and consider our general understanding and direction with the challenge of retraining our minds and not getting pulled back in the pit of counterfeit thinking. <u>There is no one who doesn't live with this struggle</u>.

The key question is:

Do you go with the flow and do not know?
Or do you strive to really see the true meaning and evaluate the situation?

_____

_____

My father reminds me that when they educate tellers at financial institutions what to look for in counterfeits bills, instead of showing them all the ways that counterfeits can occur, they'd spend their energy training them on what an authentic bill looks like. By holding up the pure authentic bill, all the counterfeits can be more easily detected. The important thing is holding up what is real and true versus what is false.

So in what area(s) of your life currently, might you be focusing on negative self-talk or thinking that is not focused on righteousness? (Counterfeit focus or unauthentic focus)

_____

_____

_____

What areas of authenticity and righteousness could you focus on to strengthen your opinions and vantage points related to this area?

_____

_____

How is your foundation built in order to achieve your destiny that God wants for you?

_____

_____

_____

What areas of your life are being influenced and encouraged to continue in the areas of counterfeit living? And how can you stop going in those directions?

_____

_____

_____

Take for example an automobile. While I'm not a petroleum expert, I know when I go to the gas pump there are usually two or three choices of fuel I can put into my car to make it run. There are three different prices and, if I have a fancy sports car, I may choose to upgrade which fuel I purchase with the scientific and engineering backing that in certain cars higher octane can burn better and more efficiently. For years, I never knew what the octane ratings meant, my focus was only on the cost. My assumption, though, is that the gas station would put gas within the pump that would make my car go.

Even as I write this, I can apply the "deconstruct to reconstruct "Revival Diet™ questioning philosophy. At my first draft of writing this, I have only the two or three choices at the pump. I know nothing about what gasoline is made of or what benefits certain choices would have. While I don't even know there are mixtures or additives in gas nor do I know what they do.

All I know is that if I want my car to go, if I want to arrive at my destination, I put my trust in the gas station to sell me what will make it run well and help get me to where I need to go and extend the life of my automobile.

Starting here with some fundamental questions that help to question my assumptions to gain new wisdom and insights goes as follows:

Why do I follow the focus of purchasing the lower-cost gasoline?

Is there any benefit to purchasing the higher octane gasoline?

Is there any detriment from purchasing the lower grade or the higher grade?

Are there any additives or ingredients that I should be aware of that may run better with my respective make and model?

Who regulates the quality of the gasoline?

Do different stations provide better quality gasoline? How would I know anything about their quality?

Do they refine gasoline differently?

Does different gasoline from various regions in the world have different vintages or short and long term affects on my automobile's functional life, performance (MPG or KPL)?

Are there storage facilities that are better than others?

In an extreme circumstance, if you filled up at one station that didn't have quality controls and regulations and they put some watered down version of gasoline that included sludge, gunk and sand, because they wanted to skimp costs and you were willing to pay the lower costs. Then later on only to find out that as you got up to cruising speed on the highway, your car started puttering and smoking and then literally ground to a halt and while you exited the car you only smelled burned and charred plastic, melted steel. At the same time, looking up the road you noticed a few other cars that appeared to have the same type of condition.

Yikes! That would not be a good day for you, your car, your insurance company, the gas station, their insurance company, the petroleum refinery company. If you chased all of them down for some answers and if the attorney's or claims adjusters had the answer "buyer beware", you'd never trust them again and for sure you'd never buy gas from that station or anyone connected to them again. The cost of that gallon of gas would skyrocket based on future repairs, replacement costs, and the time wasted in having to redo everything.

Now imagine that you need to drive that car for 10,000,000 miles over a 100 year span. If you could only use one car your entire life, and you had to fuel it and maintain it to last that whole time, would you think about the care you need to do to make it last every time you started the engine?

What parallels do you see to our bodies and nutrition from this example?

Our regulators and inspectors are there to protect us when it comes to our automobiles and many other areas in our lives. However, on the food front, there is more freedom to do whatever we want. Retraining yourself to choose out of the thousands of varieties and packages can truly be overwhelming. Especially if you are caught in the "crave it for taste" versus "craving it for the nutritional content" or for personal convenience or social acceptance or feelings of short term pleasure and excitement.

If we would rate our food intake based on an octane rating, 100 being most powerful and most nutrient packed life building foods, and 1 being garbage, where do you think we'd come in. Observations have led me to believe that the average person in the USA eats between the 20-30 ranges on the scale. Yes, I may be generous and my 'Minnesota Nice' side may be coming through or I may be inflating the curve and giving people more credit than they deserve in this scenario.

Some of the best learning comes from observation. If you want to do a qualitative study on your own, go to your average shopping mall, grocery store, around the fitness club and even around your house or your average chain restaurant and watch what fast food people are ordering and eating. Of many of the choices observed, I'd give them a 5 or 10 on the octane scale with the rounding up again as a gift.

So let's deconstruct how we get our basis (or our rationalization) for food consumption. In most cases we don't. The average person probably eats some kind of ready prepared, frozen pre-packed entry at least two out of three meals/day. (And most don't even know it) As most restaurants also only offer the packaged foods or readymade types of food that is overly salted, oiled up and created for taste.

So in the average family mom and dad works so they drop their 3-year-old at day care and their 7-year-old takes the bus to school. They ate a breakfast of high fructose corn syrup graced cereal with some packaged and sweetened yogurt, before leaving and maybe a pastry.

The 3-year-old got a snack of orange dyed goldfish, and then was given some high fructose corn syrup or sugar graced hotdogs on doubly enriched white ultra bleached buns smothered in ketchup that could send most people into diabetic shock. Upon completion the child is given a bag of juice flavored little gooey things that have *real fruit juice* added (as the 3rd or 4th ingredient). Upon further investigation there is a lot of sugar, dye and other gooey stuff mixed in to make the smiles bigger and help keep thousands of dentists buying new foreign imported cars.

At school the 7-year-old had school lunch of iceberg lettuce with a couple flakes of carrots sliced, a hamburger (fresh from the freezer on a bleached white re-enriched bun and too many other chemicals and such to list, while smothered in the ketchup (described above), a selection of tater tots (yes, they count these as a vegetable), and some chocolate pudding (who knows what is in that).

The child, after going first for the chocolate pudding, slurps it down while enjoying his chocolate milk. He then eats a couple bites of the hamburger and enjoys the tater-tots smothered in ketchup, but then gets bored with them as the student across the table enjoys his chips, he strives to negotiate a trade a tater-tot for a few chips, and does so successfully. The kid whose parents sent a healthy bag of carrots, or other vegetables, or seaweed learns to be an awesome negotiator by wheeling and dealing. It's an amazing display of unintentional consequences.

An afternoon of alternately being sluggish and hyper both kids get home to parents who are exhausted from their commute home. The parents throw in a frozen pizza and some chicken fingers drenched in high fructose corn syrup laden barbeque sauce (each respectively from the freezer with more ingredients than words on this page) and ask the kids, "How was your day?"

The kids respond like sugar junkies, saying, "Great Dad.

Are we going to be able to have some ice cream today?" The parents give in from pure exhaustion and looking for some appreciation and relief comply.

Granted, this is an extreme case, and many restaurants and fast food places have made considerable strides in the last couple years to package things a bit more healthily with better. But the fact remains, and I've witnessed this in affluent homes as well as poorer homes, that we are buying packaging ease at the expense of quality. We have supplanted cooking together with being entertained and saving time.

If you look around you may see this in so many areas of our world today; food choices, nutrition, entertainment, sports, service to others, outreach, religious organizations, media, politics, financial products, etc. So many people would rather get it in a package and not question it rather than rethink and act following God's best plan for them.

My dad used to tell me a quote he once heard somewhere that only about 5% of the people think, 20% of the people think they think, and the rest would rather die than think. When he used the word think, he was using it with the intention not only to "think" but to match the "action" with the thought as well.

To which a good friend of mine jokingly said, when I have repeated the above statistic, mentioned that about 70% of statistics are fabricated. ;)

In any case, regardless of the statistics just look around and keep your eyes opened to what, as Paul pointed out in the New Testament, about whatever is true, noble, right and pure. Focus on these.

In your life what are you just going with the flow on and accepting as normal or acceptable without really testing it?

_____

_____

_____

In what way would you test whatever you are doing to make sure it is the path you should be taking?

_____

_____

_____

_____

With the above examples of the two children and their dietary choices, what improvements do you think they could make, their parents and the schools?

_____

_____

_____

The trend that is seen in people's choices on all levels, is that they do not know how to say "no". They have not learned it, nor know what to say "no" to and what to say "go" to. But do they really have legitimate choices? Do you think they have ever really had a choice? Have they even been taught how to discern, review and to test something for worth?

Can the fault can be pointed to the parents, to the schools, to the churches, to anyone manufacturing the items, to anyone selling or marketing these items? Really? Are we just going to keep passing the blame to others?

C'mon.

No. Sorry, it's the fault of the person who puts it in their mouth.

I do believe parents have a core role to educate their children along these lines, but if they've never been told or haven't been successful at implementing, what help do they have? Seriously, some people today surveyed on various health shows and food surveys have even thought that cheese puffs are part of the dairy family... silence....gasp... jaw dropping.....
I know it leaves me completely flabbergasted, as well.

Thus the focus of retraining our approach is paramount in order to reach revival.

In both of the descriptions of the child's and parent's eating habits above and from the recent reports that more than 50% kids under the age of 18 are getting themselves set up for Type II diabetes. In my review of hundreds of periodicals and hands-on observations, the number one issue is a lack of self control.

Self-control is something that the marketing of goods is trying not to have us realize. Think of all the dollars that would be spared if people would live with more discipline, self-control, and understanding of the consequences of their decisions. In our heart of hearts we do truly know the difference between right and wrong and when we go too long in the wrong path God will graciously either move us back on course or allow us to stumble and fall. (even though it may feel like a serious cross check to our humility and pride = which we so often do indeed need.)

The Biblical angle of self-control comes from many areas. and I love the verse from Galatians 5:22-23 on the Fruit of the Spirit.

It reads: *"But the fruit of the Spirit is love, joy, peace, forbearance, kindness, goodness, faithfulness, gentleness and self-control. Against such things there is no law."*

In the past, I often misquoted the verse and call it the "Fruits" of the spirit thinking, as there were nine of them, that I could select which one I wanted to enjoy at what point in my day and that if I had love, well, I might not have gentleness, or if I have self control, I might not have joy.

Thank God for people who speak true insights and reflection that refresh and retrain me into reconstructing my understanding. A friend mentioned that it's "the fruit", not 'fruits' and that if you have one you have them all. The greatest of these is self control, which she mentioned meant that we are allowing ourselves to let God control and direct our paths.

Our attempts of self-control often only allow us to realize our limitations and our greater and deeper need for God. The self-control I'm speaking about here, that I believe the Bible emphasizes throughout, is an amazing transformational reliance on God's control in our life, (its revival in our life) and at that point then the other eight parts of the fruit are complete.

In Romans 12:2 it is written:

"Do not conform to the pattern of this world, but be transformed by the renewing of your mind. Then you will be able to test and approve what God's will is – his good, pleasing and perfect will."

John Lather, a sports researcher* has said that someone who performs something at a world class level in their respective discipline trains for at least 23 hours per week for a period of eight years to achieve that level.

That is 23 hours of high intense training for a specific activity 52 weeks per year which would be 1196 hours per year and after 8 years that would be 9568. (*noted on *15 Surprising Facts About World Class Atheletes, from* Strengthplanet.com). Most notably it was stated that the greatest determinant in top performance is time in training.

Training has been coined the greatest determinant to success. The fundamentals of the sport, the motions, the skills, the anticipation, the challenge are all helpful, but time in the training and doing them properly is where success lies.

Considering the average work week in the world is about 40 hours, we should be world class workers in just about half the amount of time in our respected profession.

The reality is that most of us are not fully engaged during those 40 hours in a week we are in at our jobs or in our profession.

This seems a bit daunting. However, what we spend our time doing becomes who we are and reflects on the world we live in.

If your calling is to be a world class athlete, good luck! You may be in the .0000001% of those who achieve such fame and fortune. I would question you, however, to consider whatever vocation God has called you in and wherever God has planted you where are to determine if you are going to be a world class "_____".

You fill in the blank(s). Either you might be a world class parent, son, Christian, spouse, professional and the list goes on of some of the inherent, sometimes seemingly tedious chores of life.

What tasks in your life would you like to become world class at?

_____

_____

_____

_____

What are you training for?

_____

_____

_____

I believe everyone is training for something. Whether you are intentional about it is another question.

The past 1.5 years I have trained about 9-18 hours per week in the area of physical fitness: running, kayaking, biking, hiking, swimming and other activities. I've run with elite Ironman and Marathon participants and often times I get into enjoyable discussions with these people on our runs of 30 minutes to 5 hours.

Those I have trained with always ask the same question, "What race are you training for?" Increasingly and with humor they are very surprised at the answer I give them, "For Christ striving to honor and support my family, my faith and my friends".

Often nodding their heads with an unsure amazement, they stutter out a "Wow! That is nice" or the most common comment is "I can't do that" or "Wow, I'm impressed, but I can't train like that unless I have a definite goal or something I am shooting for like a race on a specific date".

I am not downplaying extrinsic motivational forces that are an impetus for others to excel or sacrifice to make a training plan more meaningful. I get that without a target date or some know direction, often times the untargeted exercise route may not be as stimulating or motivating for some.

I'm sure my rationale is behind a lot of the motivation for individuals who compete in races and participate in other fitness endeavors. However I know there are a few different ways people seek fitness. To exercise or to train for something specific is one of them.

Those who train, especially for a specific race, know the discipline of certain skills that will help allow them to test their limits and develop certain muscle and repetitions that make them better at what they do.

Others who exercise may just work up a sweat and thus not test their limits but maintain good fitness, nonetheless.

The Christian Revival Diet™ values both as there is a season for all things under the heavens. However, the core philosophy is to question your intentions, your motivations, your skill set, and your competencies in order to gauge if the efforts you are engaged in are achieving the intended results you desire.

Training specifically with the proper nutrition, skill

building, practice, diet, rest, stretching, and having a gift from God to perform that activity with all your heart or for the reason you desire will lead you on a path that will be entirely unique.

For my reasons family rises to the top as well as career health and vitality. However, the main reason is still Christ at the center and to honor Him in all I do.

Over the past year and a half I've been successfully reviewing and using many structures of training and tracking, sometimes the best has been just on a small scratch sheet of paper:

Spreadsheets to track daily activities

Smart phone applications to track calories, one of the ones I like the best is the caloriecount.com, however there are many more out there as well.

Charting

Calendars

Classes

Weight tracking goals

Personal Trainers

All of these have had success. An acronym I use is POWER and I write it on a blank calendar. I write down the quantity or quality of that specific letter achieved for my workout for each day.

P = Physical & Prayerful
O = Occupational
W = Words
E = Educational
R = Rest and Recovery

Physical and Prayerful has been for me to pray as I exercise with a goal of at a minimum two hours a day with a focus on healthy nutritional eating.

Occupational has been related to my work that I at least one hour each day engaged in deepening my curiosity in my career and learning something completely new.

Words is specific to me and my aspirations in being a published writer. A famous Author, Blake, who is a friend and mentor to me, gave me some advice when I asked him how he can write over 40 books successfully in 7 years. He mentioned that he targets at least 1000 words per day. So for me to achieve the goal of having this book in print, I must at least 1000 words per day, so that is why the 'W' landed on my chart as words. Your acronym may be something else that doesn't have the POWER as mine. Again, that is ok.

Educational is related to anything else be it studying how to cook, or clean, organize better. For that matter playing my guitar or learning how to run better is all part of the educational component. For me, the goal was one new thing each day in some area.

Rest and Recovery is the hardest but when I do it the others come together with greater ease and accomplishment that even writing about it makes me yearn to do some yoga, use the foam roller to massage my legs, or to simply cuddle up under the covers.

Another acronym that I've reflected on is SPEED:

S = Sleep
P = Prayer and Physical
E = Eat Nutritionally
E = Educate Yourself
D = Dissect your performance and look for ways to improve

Another one in my office these you is:

S = Simple
C = Consistent
O = Organized
R = Repeatable
E = Energetic

Come up with an acronym that will help you to achieve the goals you desire and get closer to world class performance in whatever area God calls you to:

_____

_____

_____

_____

_____

_____

_____

_____

_____

_____

_____

_____

Journal a summary of what you have done for one whole day. Thoughts, habits, food, viewing, connections, everything. Deconstruct it and reconstruct it one thing at a time.

_____

_____

_____

_____

_____

———————————————————

———————————————————

———————————————————

———————————————————

———————————————————

———————————————————

———————————————————

———————————————————

———————————————————

What is the acronym for the life you've let happen to you?

———————————————————

———————————————————

———————————————————

———————————————————

Mine personally was LAZY

L = Letting it happen
A = Angst
    (The German word for worry, tension and anxiety)
Z = Zeal
Y = Youthful

Letting it happen was a mantra that I felt I was doing in many areas. Rather than being intentional I was just kind of going with the motions.

Angst would sometimes lead to a bitterness and frustration as to why I am not achieving what I want to, and in some cases an apathy that fueled greater negative thinking.

Zeal for the world would be part of what I strived to do, however my intentions would be to receive accolades or appreciation versus doing it to the Lord.

Youthful lack of maturity and proper thinking would

sometimes cloud my thinking and lead to selfishness and improper rational thinking about the situation or issue I was dealing with. I tried to find the solution on my terms instead of on God's terms. The quote comes to mind, "Youth is often wasted on the young". I don't know who said it, but a gentleman who was my boss once said that to me often when I was eager to do things without really thinking it through or focusing in the most rational way.

Where in your life will you renew and stop conforming?

_____

_____

_____

_____

_____

_____

Don't let your work in God take the place of God working in you. What are you working for in Christ that might be better to just allow God to work in you?

_____

_____

_____

5
REENERGIZE

"Come near to God and He will come near to you. Wash your hands, you sinners, and purify your hearts, you double-minded. Grieve, mourn and wail. Change your laughter to mourning and your joy to gloom. Humble yourselves before the Lord, and He will lift you up."
James 4:8-10

"For in my inner being I delight in God's law; but I see another law at work in me, waging war against the law of my mind and making me a prisoner of the law of sin at work within me. What a wretched man I am! Who will rescue me from this body that is subject to death?"
Romans 7:22-24

"Forgive, forget and move forward with faith!"

I love this saying above, and I love this verse below...

"Therefore, I urge you, brothers and sisters, in view of God's mercy, to offer your bodies as a living sacrifice, holy and pleasing to God – this is your true and proper worship. Do not conform to the pattern of this world, but be transformed by the renewing of your mind. Then you will be able to test and approve what God's will is – His good, pleasing and perfect will. Romans 12:1-2

You will stumble, you will slip, you will falter, forces will push against you that try to thwart your destiny, and there are days when you will fail. However with God's we can keep pressing forward no matter what happens.

"Forgive, forget, and move forward with faith!"

I have said this often sometimes, and I sometimes add *'repent, confess, turn from my sin and keep my eyes on Jesus.'*

Really the question we should ask it, "What do we have to move forward with?" I keep thinking 'with God' is the simple and the only answer.

What great words to consider and to live by, but so hard to implement in your life.

When we feel wronged, we must come to understand that it wasn't fully intentional, or we may be reading into it more than we should. We must remember that people do things for their own reasons, not ours. When someone has affected us in a negative manner. If we really check our emotions, and interpret the situation correctly, and look at the facts and discern if our emotional side has warranted this interpretation of the situation. Looking back we often find we were wrong.

Deconstruct your emotions. What exactly are you feeling? Can you fully comprehend all the emotions and the thoughts you have at one time?

The refreshing thing in my life is that I've found that 99.9 times out of 100, the things that I think might go wrong, end of never occurring. When something does indeed go wrong, it is usually my fault! Although these are sometimes tough lessons to learn, I earnestly need to get more serious about learning and accepting my responsibility in the minor percentage.

My responsibility is often to get myself out of God's way and keep my eyes on where He is going and what He is doing versus tripping over myself and running into the proverbial brick walls.

Reflect on your life up until now:

What are some of the items in your life that have caused you fear, anxiety, second guessing, or anxiousness? And how often did what you imagined actually occurred? What have you done to overcome this?

Proverbs 3:5-6 *"Trust in the Lord with all your heart, lean not on your own understanding; in all your ways acknowledge Him and He will make your paths straight."*

This was the first Bible verse I ever memorized. It sums up so much and helps you adjust your thinking and align your focus to where it needs to be.

How many of the things that did happen badly in your life actually weren't part of what you did wrong?

_____

_____

_____

_____

_____

How many things were surprises above? What will you do about them? (Better question... How will you seek God's direction and allow Him to move forward?)

_____

_____

_____

_____

_____

I am speaking about your personal responsibility for your actions and your life. Yes, there are certain things that occur that are completely not your fault. However, it's always your choice how you react to them and how you manage to persevere through the trial you are facing.

As a parent, it's so much easier to see when our children point to others as the cause of their pain or frustration, when it really is so clear that it's their irrationality or fact, then for us to see it when we do it. The hard thing is for us is to rationally admit our wrong doings.

Galatians 6:5 highlights:
"For each will have to bear his own load". And in Colossians 3:23 *"Whatever you do, work heartily, as for the Lord and not for men."*

So reenergize with the focus of whatever your situation may be. That you are able to focus 100% at following through to completion on the task God has given you to perform with courage, humility and love.

Relating to the healthy-focus of the revival diet, I hope you have started to understand that it's not about just losing weight, or eating right, or doing some little tasks, but living right for

Christ in all things.

What have you done to reenergize? To be fully engaged? To be revived?

_____

_____

_____

_____

"Therefore, I urge you, brothers and sisters, in view of God's mercy, to offer your bodies as a living sacrifice, holy and pleasing to God – this is your true and proper worship. Do not conform to the pattern of this world, but be transformed by the renewing of your mind. Then you will be able to test and approve what God's will is – his good, pleasing and perfect will. Romans 12:1-2

We all have tried to do things as band aids to keep us happy, but end up feeling more and more empty. Some of the negative things might be excessive eating, drink excessive energy drinks, excessive abstinence from eating, too much caffeine, sugar or other to be reenergized. Basically this includes anything that might control you that you say "I've got to have it or I can't live without it".

Some may start a new training schedule or routine, buying something new, moving somewhere, starting a new diet, some may engage in sinful activity or some other fad related thing all to alleviate whatever pain or emptiness they may have.

God wants us to find his balance in Him.

Where does God want you to find balance in your life?

_____

_____

_____

_____

What negative actions might be lingering in your life that you could ask God's providence to heal you from?

_____

_____

_____

For three years I asked a group of friends to pray for me regarding balance. Their prayers eventually paid off. But in the end I realized that no matter what my situation was "I" could not find it. My prayer should have been to ask God to grant me a peace and a balance, that which only He could provide.

"Rejoice in the Lord always. I will say it again: Rejoice! Let your gentleness be evident to all. The Lord is near. Do not be anxious about anything, but in everything, by prayer and petition, with Thanksgiving, present your requests to God. And the peace of God, which transcends all understanding, will guard your hearts and your minds in Christ Jesus."

Philippians 4:4-7

Finding God's peace and getting 100% reenergized is found through this simple equation:

Connections with God = Following Jesus in all things...He is peace

Which may include ...

Daily studying the Bible and praying to God
+
Giving of our self to Him & to others in service
+
Repenting of our sins
+
Fellowship with other Christians
+
Serving where God wants us to
+

Turning from temptations
+
Forgiving others who
have wronged you

As you read God's Holy word, reflect on what other things you could add that would grant you greater relationship and connection with God. Anytime I read the Bible I ask myself these questions:

Regarding Philippians 4:4-7, please answer these questions below:

What does it say about God? What can I learn from the context?

_____

_____

_____

What does it say that applies to you? (either to do or consider)

_____

_____

_____

What can you apply to your life today? And how can you engage this learning in your life?

_____

_____

_____

Please take out your Bible and read the following verses and jot down what comes to mind after you read and reflect:
1) What does the section of scripture say?
2) What does it mean?
3) How can I apply it to my life?
4) And any other good application to your life?

Romans 10:17 *How often are you reading Christ's word?*

_____

_____

_____

_____

_____

1 John 1:9 *What sins do you need to confess?*

_____

_____

_____

_____

John 3:16-17 *What did God give to show He loved us? Why did He do that?*

_____

_____

_____

_____

John 13:1-7 *Whose feet have you washed?*

_____

_____

_____

_____

Mark 12:28-34 *What is the greatest commandment? How are you living it out?*

_____

_____

_____

Knowing Christ is our peace is such an amazing and awesome privilege. He is the source of everything as it all was made by Him and through Him, and He holds all things together. Knowing this is at the center of all things. Knowing that He is where the source of our everything, truly refreshes my soul.

Colossians 1:16-20:
"For in him all things were created: things in heaven and on earth, visible and invisible, whether thrones or powers or rulers or authorities; all things have been created through him and for him.

He is before all things, and in Him all things hold together. And He is the head of the body, the church; He is the beginning and the firstborn from among the dead, so that in everything He might have the supremacy. For God was pleased to have all His fullness dwell in Him, and through Him to reconcile to himself all things, whether things on earth or things in heaven, by making peace through His blood, shed on the cross."

Christ is the revival.

Christ is balance.

Christ is love.

Christ is leadership.

There is a direct correlation between the more revival we witness in our world with how much more each individual believer opens up to allow Christ to work in their lives in every instance.

The more God's people humble themselves and pray, the more revival grows through every person, to every family, to every office, and every school bus and every playground, and every community -- eventually completely filling our world.

I wish I could say it is as easy as setting new goals and changing your attitude, or some simple kind of seven steps to some kind of success, some type of habits, buying something new or doing something to reenergize you. While those may give a temporary satisfaction for that which is perishing in comparison to that which is eternal, the reality it is all by His power!

So in what ways will you strive to plug into God's energy in your life to recharge?

_____

_____

_____

_____

Try documenting everything you eat for 14 days in a row on some tracking method (either your calendar, sending emails to yourself, a journal, or something). Keep track of your food intake, activities, and how you fell.

After those 14 days describe how you feel here:

_____

_____

_____

_____

_____

_____

_____

Coming back to our five senses: Sound, sight, taste, smell,

touch. If our lives could only encompass these five areas, life would be purely experiential; however, when we bring the blessings of emotions into the situation, we end up having literally hundreds of combinations of feelings that affect our moods, our health, and our interactions.

Some of the emotions we encounter are:

Fear, loneliness, sorrow, sadness, joy, pain, fatigue, sluggishness, anger, engagement, pride, jealously, rage, hunger, satisfaction, satiation, desire, compassion, lust, greed, graciousness, confusion, loss, grief, unfulfilled expectations, determination, arrogance, and so many more.

The challenge again is feeling and knowing what we are going through related to our senses and our emotions and how it affects our situation in the world.

What can we do about it?

So often the problem stems from our inability to rationalize the situation and base it on facts in order to react in a manner that enhances our walk with God.

H.A.L.T. an acronym for Hungry, Angry, Lonely or Tired, is an acronym that my wife stuck up on the refrigerator. Her Mothers of Preschool group gave a lecture on it which is a great reminder to us in stressful times. H.A.L.T. first and think about these questions: Are they acting up or emotionally falling apart because of their hunger, anger, loneliness, tired? This was a good checkpoint when our kids were under seven years old. However, I'd amend this and add H.A.L.T. & C.O.G., with the C.O.G. equal to 'Centered on God'.

If one is centered on God there will be a gift of rationalism and perspective that brings an open acceptance of understanding and relevance towards whatever comes our way. When this is not present, then the irrational reality demands a different approach.

I bring this up as it's an example of how to deal with people and situations that affect our current reality. The amazing thing is that as you can see it in your children easily, again the focus of realizing it in yourself is very difficult and just when you need it the most is when you probably won't see it. Adults need to H.A.L.T. more than even the kids do in the activities of their lives.

When do you see times when the wheels fall off of your endeavors (faith, family, relational, emotional, occupational, etc.)?

_____

_____

_____

_____

_____

What are some examples recently in relationships, work, family, friends where things went bad?

_____

_____

_____

_____

_____

What could you do to better center yourself on God (H.A.L.T & C.O.G.) to find the strength and power to achieve results for Him in this area?

_____

_____

_____

Where in your life are you still living in sin? And how will you break free from this sin? What do you need to confess, repent, and turn from?

_____

_____

_____

_____

_____

_____

You may ask, why I keep asking these question about sin? Well, sin is the greatest barrier you face?

I'll ask you, 'Do we as humans easily repeat the same sins?' 'Some even that we are not sure we are doing?' 'Does it really hurt us to refresh our soul and or direction?' (If you need greater support or help please consult your pastor, a Biblical counselor, or other accountability partners)

Are you standing strong in Christ against your sins?

"No temptation has seized you except what is common to man. And God is faithful, He will not let you be tempted beyond what you can bear."

1 Corinthians 10:13

How has God been faithful in your trials or temptations?

_____

_____

_____

_____

_____

6
REGRET NO MORE

"For God did not send his Son into the world to condemn the world, but to save the world through Him."
John 3:17

"What can Jesus save us from?", a friend of mine who is a skeptic asks me often.

My answer is that He can save us from eternal hell and eternal separation from God's love. That's it. Either you want this eternal saving grace or the consequences.

Next topic.

"The doctor of the future will give no medicine, but will interest his patient in the care of the human frame, in diet and in the cause and prevention of disease"
Thomas Jefferson

Sorry, all you physicians and 'health care' providers out there. The profession, I've heard some people say, might be better named 'the sick care industry'. Your secret is out of the bag. Let's be real. In so many ways you are stuck in a reactive role and I don't fault you individually. Your esteemed job shows cracks in the foundation when you have zero or one nutritional course to graduate. I'm not contesting that your job doesn't hold merit.

I believe it is a very worthy profession and holds an important role fills a much needed place. But, just like every person on earth and in every career, the biggest room in anyone's house is the room for improvement.

However, as the ignorance of most people allows the belief that you are the source of health and positive coaching, i.e. as a Health Care Provider, are you really in the health care field, or is it the disease care field, working as a disease care provider? Most physicians working with their patients are in a reactive mode with prescriptions as their healing diagnosis, which often lead to more complications. Some do know what could have been done to prevent it, but would the patients have listened and acted upon it, or do they have time to even educate the patients?

How many physicians have simply given up on asking people to change their lives in order to live healthier?

I've also spoke to many physicians, who have openly admitted we prescribe medications because most people will not make the healthy life changes needed to improve their health. They've said they don't have time to teach someone who isn't willing to change. I agree with them in the latter part.

Most physicians follow this approach as they have been trained to prescribe medicine (I'll excuse them as it's not their choice, realistically it is more the system that promotes this mentality, and each consumer who buys into it is as well just as guilty even if ignorantly mislead – no excuses):

Illness = Check up/limited physical i.e. quick problem focused analysis (tongue out, look @ eyes, check problems and ears) + Drug prescription + Don't change your life.

Some of the warning side effects listed for taking the prescriptions are downright lunacy. …..this medicine may cause drowsiness, loss of hair, kidney failure, heart attack, if you have a stroke please discontinue use… Can they really say by listing these effects during an ocean cinematography shot of a healthy person dancing on a beach, that they are preparing people for the reality of using their drug? Who are they kidding? We'll, the corporate coffers that manufacture the drugs and the millions and millions of people who start down prescription row follow the crowd.

Simply put, the buyer must be consciously aware and engaged in all aspects of purchases and use. Shouldn't the buyer beware in all purchases or investments of time, relationally or otherwise?

Please jot down what your last visit to the health care provider was like. Were there any questions or comments about nutrition, sleep, exercise or other things they prompted you to become healthier?

_____

_____

_____

_____

_____

Like the quote from Thomas Jefferson says about the doctor of the future prescribing nutrition to prevent disease, proper nutrition can be an important factor healing. When you really deconstruct the big picture you see the issue is disease. We are in a sinful nature with a planned obsolescence and expiration date, which no one knows the day or the time.

Some of the diseases are in our control and full influence on our illness, some of us get sick without our true choice or limited participation. However, we all own 100% of the attitude we relate to and how we learn, discern and apply what we need to do. Our doctor may know how to treat disease. But must discern, trust and verify what the approach we use and how we handle these issues.

This is simply another area in our lives where revival is ultimately called for.

Illness = Drug Prescription or procedure when needed
        + Action and Joy (1 Thes. 5:16)
            + a Holistic Diet review i.e.
        (that includes a nutritional analysis, lifestyle analysis, health and physical assessment, sleep review, relational and emotional check in and a spiritual well being review)

If you could take a snapshot of what some people do in a 24-hour period you could see a glimpse of why they are in the a less than healthy state. Now compound those activities over 365 days for however many years they have been doing these things.

So often you hear the person say, "I just don't know how it happened?!?!?"

Their destiny is fulfilled. Their lazy ignorance became their excuse du jour, which ends like a surprise.

What bad habits do you have that have landed you @ your destiny?

I never knew my biological grandfather. I was not even born when he passed away. He left my mom, her four brothers, and his wife. What a tragedy that could have been avoided.

He died when my mom was 17 at the age of 34. He died from emphysema from excessive smoking. The cigarettes controlled him to a rapid death that he couldn't break free from. He basically killed himself even after the diagnosis, and the doctor's stern warning to change his lifestyle. I never really understood what that affect must have had on my mom and aunts and uncles growing up.

The reality and the blessing that came out of that was that my mom and dad's health and influences has changed due to those situations, which also changed me and prayerfully my children as well.

How many other potential ills, deaths, feelings of lackluster living, and joyless 'going through the motions' could be avoided if lifestyle changes were made? Anything from your past?

_____

_____

_____

_____

I was blessed because by the time I was born my grandmother remarried an amazing Christian man who I have always known as my grandpa. God bless his soul for loving me and the other grandchildren like they were his own. I have been blessed to have so many awesome memories as a child with him.

My father was diagnosed with two things recently. High blood pressure and high triglycerides. Upon the doctor's diagnosis and prescription, my dad said that he is not taking the medicines. First he wanted to make a lifestyle change. He came home and starting breaking apart his diet, reinvigorating his exercise, and looking for where these two areas of illness could stem from.

He read books and took action to change. The two areas were caused, my dad thought from his research, on sugars sweets, and saturated fats from meats. Ironically, the doctor had no clue on what my dad could change in his life. That doctor only had medications, full of side effects, to dole out.

Researching all the causes of these two ailments, my father wrote down a list of what causes could influence this and then went to work.

Potential Causes of High Triglycerides (*source webmd.com*)

Eating too much fat and sugary foods
High blood sugar
Obesity
Underactive Thyroid
Regularly eating more calories than you burn
Excessive alcohol drinking

Potential Solutions

Stay at a healthy weight
Limit fats and sugars in your diet
Be more active
Limit alcohol and don't smoke

Potential Causes of High Blood Pressure (*Source webmd.com*)

Smoking
Being overweight or obese
Too much salt in the diet
Lack of physical activity
Older age
Stress
Too much alcohol consumption
Adrenal and thyroid disorders

Potential solutions

DASH (Dietary Approaches to Stop Hypertension) diet
Lose weight
Limit salt and exercise more
Reduce alcohol consumption
Eating healthy foods

Here is how he monitored the two areas to do what he needed to achieve success:

Monitor blood pressure

Track food and <u>don't</u> eat the foods that are causing the issue.

Now let's put this in perspective. At age 76 it is hard to change your habits. He went to work and made these changes and within less than 30 days, he was back to healthy levels on these two areas.

The coup d'état on high triglycerides and high blood pressure was first strategically analyzed, then action followed with prayer, a journal of vitals was tracked and inventoried on a daily basis. The goal was managed and inspected and the discipline of my father led the revolt and revival needed to change his lifestyle to avoid the medications.

Upon returning to the physician and subsequent tests, the proverbial "jaw dropped Doc", just asked in amazement: "What did you do to change these tests so fast? I have never seen any such changes occur so rapidly ever in my career."

My father told him.

The doctor didn't believe him and asked him for a second set of tests.

If a 76 year old can have this kind of success, what about a 16 year old? What about a 33 year old? A 50 year old? Or 60 year old?

So many people just take their diagnosis and just settle for less in health related areas of their lives while medicating the issue. They seek the quick fix drug, technology or medical advice first instead of prayer, action and lifestyle change.

This analysis can be used to not only diagnose but also about how to cure a malady you have. As well as with the focus that encompasses improving a strength that you have, and a gift

God has given for you.

Take another example of this: One of my friends and running buddies, who runs a strong 7 minute 30 second mile over long distances. He took on the task for to break the 7 minute mile area. He did the same as my dad did. He set his goal, prayed about it, sought advice and new research, started tracking actions, and took action to achieve that. Within 6 months he now can run a sustained 6 minute 30 second mile. That is a huge breakthrough for my friend who is in his 40s.

I did the same, lowering my speed from about 8 minute miles in 2011 to 7 minute mile in 2012. Then I surprised myself on a 5k in 2013 running at a personal record at 6:10 per minute mile over the 5k distance at age 42. Whatever your time or goal is, I'd recommend you striving toward it.

You may ask the question, where do I go to find the resources to learn and get the advice needed? I found if I first bring it to prayer, then God guides me and puts the resources in front of me, it may be through a friend, a book, a coach, an advisor, going to your local library and investing in some research.

"Forgetting what lies behind and straining forward to what lies ahead, I press on toward the goal for the prize of the upward call of God in Christ Jesus." Philippians 3:13-14

What can you press on with in your life today?

_____

_____

_____

Isn't knowing that God has great things for you refreshing? Please don't ever forget His promises.

"For I know the plans I have for you," declares the Lord, "plans to prosper you and not to harm you, plans to give you hope and a future." Jeremiah 29:11

What plans does Christ have for you today?

_____

_____

_____

_____

_____

In light of the above verses and thoughts, take some notes in the following pages.

What areas of greater strength do you believe God wants you to enhance?

_____

_____

_____

_____

_____

What do you need to forget about and move forward with?

_____

_____

_____

_____

_____

What is holding you back from your goals?

_____

_____

_____

_____

_____

What could you track daily to see if you are on the right path?

_____

_____

_____

_____

What have you failed in consistently that you can find a partner to support you in? To balance out your weaknesses?

_____

_____

_____

What have you succeeded in amazingly that others call a great strength of yours? How can you use it daily to help serve others?

_____

_____

_____

The greatest determinant in success in just about any endeavor is your ability to train for that goal. So, how are you practicing for your goals? If you write your goals down but do nothing to move forward towards them, you will never achieve your goal. You have vision and a direction but no muscle to get

you there but as a friend, Philip, used to say, 'Vision without implementation is hallucination'.

The reality is when you reflect on your true performance,

every effort can be reflected on in light of what you are striving for. The hard dilemma is that often we may be just going through the motions. We are competent, but not excellent. We can do it, but our heart isn't 100% into it. Doing your best and striving for excellence when you practice as well as you perform is the key no matter what you do. So both practice and performance can help you achieve your direction. And the majority of the time you will be practicing.

From Wikipedia:

Practice
noun

Repeated exercise in or performance of an activity or skill so as to acquire or maintain proficiency in it.

Perform (an activity) or exercise (a skill) repeatedly or regularly in order to improve or maintain one's proficiency.

Consider these questions:

In what areas are you just going through the motions?

_____

_____

_____

How can you break through your current plateau for greater success?

_____

_____

_____

What might be holding you back from achieving the success you desire?

_____

_____

_____

Which people in your life can you give you advice, positive encouragement or motivational support to help you achieve your goal?

_____

_____

_____

How are you practicing in order to raise your level of spiritual strength?

_____

_____

What else are your training or practicing for?

_____

_____

How can you break through your current plateau for greater success?

_____

_____

_____

_____

What prayer do you need to pray now?

_____

_____

_____

_____

7

REMEMBER AND REPENT

"²⁰ My son, pay attention to what I say;
turn your ear to my words.
²¹ Do not let them out of your sight,
keep them within your heart;
²² for they are life to those who find them
and health to one's whole body.
²³ Above all else, guard your heart,
for everything you do flows from it.
²⁴ Keep your mouth free of perversity;
keep corrupt talk far from your lips.
²⁵ Let your eyes look straight ahead;
fix your gaze directly before you.
²⁶ Give careful thought to the paths for your feet
and be steadfast in all your ways.
²⁷ Do not turn to the right or the left;
keep your foot from evil."

Proverbs 4:20-27

For about 400 years the Israelites wandered in the desert, at some point the people thought this was their eternity. For some of their generations, it may have seemed like their whole earthly life was wandering, which it literally was for many of them. Their lives were like going in a circle, wandering in a barren landscape with no place to call their permanent home. They were nomads wandering around their homes were constantly being pulled out as they relied on God for their next steps and followed a cloud by day and pillar of fire at night. (While collecting manna, grumbling, bickering and complaining).

Was the wandering prescribed to them to remember how they wandered? Was it to rid the captive mentality post their slavery in Egypt? Was it prescribed for their complete and utter reliance on God in their lives? Many people have speculated and have theories about why they wandered. In either case we remember today that God is sovereign and His reason is still being played out today as we study and apply these lessons to our lives and in our own wandering.

Proverbs 4:26, from the previous page, focuses on *"Give careful thought to the paths for your feet and be steadfast in all your ways."* In my life, I haven't often given careful thought and I have not always been steadfast in all my ways.

Another way I've heard this verse described is *"Ponder the paths of your feet, make steadfast your way with the Lord"*. This verse happens to be one of my life verses. Although so many times when I was younger, I rarely followed the guidance or pondered the path of my feet.

This verse has since carried me through my walk as I choose which foods I should eat, what to watch on TV, what books to read, what radio stations we listen to, how to have meaningful relationships and then, as it has become more and more refining in helping me achieve my goals, has helped me make choices with God that have better outcomes in many other areas. I wandered myself, and I learned along the way, but it wasn't and isn't the best way to learn.

What times in your life have you been successful in considering your paths?

_____

_____

_____

_____

What trends do you see in these times?

_____

_____

_____

What can catapult you more in that direction?

_____

_____

_____

What do you need to do yourself? What can you ask Christ to help you with? Who can you ask to pray for you?

_____

_____

_____

_____

Where have you wandered in your life?

_____

_____

_____

Consider this question:

In what areas of your life did you not give careful thought and what were the good and bad outcomes?

_____

_____

Regarding nutritional choices you could perhaps spend one or two days tracking everything that enters your mouth. I personally spent 3.5 months doing this, and I was amazed at the wisdom and strength it provided me in my choices.

At one time, I heard a sermon that spoke about fasting, and the focus of not having anything in our life that "controls" us, or that we could show addictive behavior towards.

For some people this could be chocolate, sugar, coffee, alcohol, spicy foods, or sugary foods. For some people it could be lack of purpose, sexual sin, emotional sin, judgmental pride, financial sin and many other possibilities. While I follow the mantra of having everything in balance, I wanted to make sure that nothing controlled me. For me it was sugar that I found hard to break free from.

What controls you that you can't go without?

_____

_____

_____

_____

I was 14 years old when my Dad and I went on a canoe trip down the Namekogen and the St. Croix rivers in Wisconsin. On day three, he had to leave me at the campsite and hitch hike into town to get his fix of coffee, as he'd forgotten to pack it in the canoe, and the searing headache he had was debilitating. That was an experience that is etched in my mind, for not being able to function without something controlling you. My mom edited this part and wrote in the side bar that she's glad I didn't use her similar situation when we were traveling around Austria together when I was in college.

My father was somewhat bound or controlled by caffeine and my commitment has to strive to never have something or someone other than Christ have that controlling and limiting power in my life. Recently, he has kicked the caffeine habit. A man of determination and steadfast persistence. Great work Papa E!

But dealing with sugar my wife and I and three boys determined not to eat anything sugary for lent this past year. It was tough, but then we decided that every time we were offered something sweet, we would take it and put it in the freezer. We ended up with a laundry-basket sized load of sweets over that time period. Just imagining that hadn't we given it up, we would have consumed that amount of sugar and other junk makes me ill and really question what it does to your body?

Whatever amount of reflection and study you put into your journey, whether for a day or 120 days, please jot down what new insights you've learned from doing this. What foods can you go without?

_____

_____

_____

What things can you go without?

_____

_____

_____

What may control you in your life?

_____

_____

_____

What sins can you go without?

_____

_____

_____

Please read and reflect on these verses and please jot down what application you can have on your life:

Colossians 3:2: *Where should you set your mind?*

_____

_____

_____

_____

Psalm 1:1-6: *Who is blessed? What do they do and what don't they do?*

_____

_____

_____

_____

Matthew 6:33: *What should we seek first?*

_____

_____

_____

_____

2 Timothy 2:15: How should you handle God's truth?

_____

_____

_____

_____

Romans 8:5: What is your mind focused on?

_____

_____

_____

_____

Matthew 6:24: What or who are you serving?

_____

_____

_____

_____

Proverbs 4:25: What are you looking at?

_____

_____

_____

_____

1 Peter 3:17: When should you suffer?

_____

_____

_____

_____

1 Corinthians 10:13: What temptation has seized you?

_____

_____

_____

_____

Philippians 4:8: Where are your thoughts?

_____

_____

_____

_____

2 Timothy 3:16-17: What is the word of God to be used for and why?

Ecclesiastes 9:10 : Where are you doing?

_____

_____

_____

_____

Proverbs 2:2-5: How and where are you prayerfully searching wisdom?

_____

_____

_____

Colossians 2:6-8: How world Christ rate your worldly view? Are you centered on Him or the world?

_____

_____

_____

Philippians 4:13: What can you do in Christ?

_____

_____

_____

1 Peter 2:1-25: What should you rid yourself of? What should you crave?

_____

_____

_____

Romans 12:9: How shall we love?

_____

_____

_____

_____

James 1:1-27: So much…. What can you apply?

_____

_____

_____

Proverbs 15:20: How can you apply this to your life?

_____

_____

_____

1 Corinthians 13:11: A child or an adult: where are you in your spiritual walk?

_____

_____

_____

Hebrews 12:1-2: What sin holds you back? What can you throw off? Where to keep your gaze?

_____

_____

_____

1 John 2:1-29: So much ….. What can you apply?

_____

_____

_____

_____

Titus 2:11-12: How shall we live?

_____

_____

_____

_____

Proverbs 18:7: How shall you guard your lips?

_____

_____

_____

_____

Matthew 24:13: How long will you need to stand firm?

_____

_____

_____

_____

Proverbs 6:6-8: The ant? How can that relate to you?

_____

_____

_____

_____

Philippians 3:9-14: How shall we strive?

_____

_____

_____

John 3:16-17: Why did Jesus die?

_____

_____

_____

_____

Luke 17:1-37: Wow! Application?

_____

_____

_____

_____

Romans 1:12: Encourage each other

_____

_____

_____

_____

Proverbs 16:3: What plans shall you commit to the Lord?

_____

_____

_____

_____

1 Thessalonians 5:21-22: What should you test? What should you avoid?

_____

_____

_____

_____

1 John 3:16: What is love?

_____

_____

Proverbs 8:35: What do you receive if you find Christ?

_____

_____

_____

_____

Psalm 119:1-2: Who is blessed?

_____

_____

_____

_____

Proverbs 5:9: What to avoid? What to embrace?

_____

_____

_____

_____

Psalm 32:8: Who will teach you?

_____

_____

_____

_____

Luke 9:62: Who is fit to serve?

_____

_____

_____

_____

Psalm 119:105: What is God's word?

_____

_____

_____

_____

Psalm 25:7-21: What application could you have?

_____

_____

_____

_____

Psalm 48:14: Who is God? What will He be?

_____

_____

_____

Now review these past 41 verses and consider what overall could you do today?

_____

_____

_____

_____

_____

It's the start that counts and the next few steps along the way.

I find in my own exercising it's all in the first 90 seconds, and really it boils down to the first 3 seconds.

Let's face it, it's all about the start. Some people say showing up is all you have to do. However, I think it's about the start. I can drive to the fitness club and do nothing. But once I begin and put my energy and focus on something, my chances of finishing go up exponentially. Try it, you will see.

When I commit and start moving through the first 3 seconds it gets easier. Then after the first 90 seconds it is even easier. I realize that the greatest challenge is that which is my mind, so the positive mantra is just get me through the next second. Once I tell myself that then after that the next 60-90 minutes fly by.

Swimming has not been something that comes naturally to me. The water is cold, and outside of splashing on warm sunny beaches, originally my thoughts were on "why spend time swimming laps in cold water?"

Well, out at Lake Okoboji about one mile across from Arnold's Park, I left my aunt and uncles cabin and decided to swim. I put on my wetsuit, and walked down to the dock. On the way, I heard from people, "Are you really going?", "Please be safe", "Don't go there, it'll be better just to walk", "How are you going to have a marker so people see you?" Within the first 30 seconds of my deciding to go, before I even left the house, everyone was trying to steer me from my goal, by trying to make me worried. Their negative self-talk was trying to hold me back.

Upon entering the water, everything in my mind was saying, "maybe they are right", but then my counter point was mentioning "keep going, keep going, keep going". After the next 60 seconds in the water, as my body started getting use to the cold, I felt completely free and supercharged. The next 90 minutes flew by as I paddled through the fresh water. The streaming lines of sun glowing through the clouds as I enjoyed the physical challenge.

I did tie a blaze orange life vest that floated about seven feet behind me as a buoy so boaters could see me in the water from afar. So, some of the forewarning and caution was helpful.

Before that outdoor swim I set a New Year's goal was to swim 100 miles in 1 year. I figured that would be 2 miles/week for 50 weeks. With my background that would be painful, as a soccer and hockey player, swimming has never been a forte of mine. Prior to that year I think I probably swam less than 1 mile/year without ever counting the laps.

So I tracked it on a sheet by the quarter mile, with each quarter mile about 18 lengths.

The first mile I did took me about 1 hour and 20 minutes. I was exhausted. Over the course of that year, I started to become more efficient, and mixed in with my longer mile workouts were various ½ and ¾ mile workouts. By June my 1 mile time dropped to 50 minutes. That was quite a nice adaptation and improvement. By the end of July my time had improved even more to about 40 minutes, and to my amazement I was able to achieve the 100 miles 4+ months earlier than the target goal. I finished on my mom's birthday in August. That week I swam an extra 2 miles to finish on that day, often times swimming on my lunch hour as well. I think I totaled about 6 miles that week to cram it in.

I read that many of the elite athletes doing long distance races don't focus on the race through the process, they only focus on the next step or the next 100 feet, a tree on a hill, or whatever they set before them as a marker.

Some things that God puts in your path are so you will learn that you can only rely on Him and follow Him one step at a time. Similar to the wandering Moses endured.

Raising kids is much the same, and God forces you to trust Him. He forces you to think 18-25 years later to make investments in your children's education if it were a simple roadmap without detours, trials, tests and their own personality development, it wouldn't be as adventurous, and it wouldn't be something that you'd be forced to completely rely on God in your life for.

So remembering how to break through for the first 3 to 90 seconds is vital. I believe it's mental and spiritual. As the mental mindset can compel you to victory, the spiritual side can ground you for the realities facing you. Whatever time line it takes you to break through, know it and knowing yourself is important. If you can build a resilience and strength for getting through the next 90 seconds, you can do it. I personally use positive self-talk or Bible verses, mantras and viewpoints to help strengthen me in my daily duties, ranging from sleeping, eating, waking, cleaning, organizing, moving, working and so much more. I've added a list of my favorites in the appendix as they keep growing as I write this.

What personal mantra have you used to get you through the first 90 seconds?

Personally one of my greatest struggles is having consistency and being self-disciplined, especially when it comes to following through to mastery on a certain project or discipline. One of these is sleep and rest.

For me, the fear of missing something in life propels me to want to be involved in everything and attentive to everything but I know I can't.

As a young child, going over to a friend's house for a sleepover meant me wanting to stay up the whole night, no matter the cost. On one occasion, there were about 15 kids at a birthday party and only 2-3 of us managed not to sleep. We were about 10/11 years old, and I always stayed awake the longest.

That desire has not left me as I've aged. But there is a cost. I am sometimes not as sharp nor able to focus mentally as I could. I have also made some bad decisions spiritually and rationally without the proper sleep.

I wasn't aware until recently that most of the metabolic functions that our bodies performs happens when we sleep. These metabolic functions help repair, strengthen, feed and prepare our bodies for good health.

Thus, sleeping helps the body, soul, and mind, but for me it's hard to have enough self-discipline to get to bed on time. It has been more of an "all or nothing". Staying awake until I crash and then getting up, which if I am striving for peak performance, has not been beneficial as my body has not been able to heal and repair itself to the level that it needs. (And sometimes even my wife will notice and remind me that I didn't get much sleep to be alert and functional).

Remember from chapter two doing your body scan. Every night and every morning if you do a body/mind/soul scan you will be much healthier as you will know what you need to remember and what you need to forget. As well in knowing yourself it will be vital as you assess what it is you are call to do today.

One of the best weeks I had was when I prayed and meditated on God's word throughout the whole day. Following this type of schedule, everything went awesome. Even when the challenges arrived that I had to face, I was alert, well rested and ready for God-centered action:

You've heard people speak about a model week. A week pre-planned that they accomplish what they set out to do, and have the hours and days filled with the proper items in order to achieve their goals.

This is where I recommend tracking on your calendar on a given day what it is you accomplished or intend to accomplish. We spoke earlier about doing a body scan. Other types of scans could be a schedule scan, work scan, relationship scan, goal scan, sin scan, emotional scan, or financial scan. Yes, you see, holistically there are a ton of areas that growth could occur. Again holding the lens of God up to these items will increase effectiveness for Him. While doing it you will see and reflect on what you could do better.

> For me my ideal day would include the following:
> Exercise (mental, physical, spiritual)
> Time with family
> Time alone
> Time listening to sermons and God's word
> Working efficient and hard @ work
> Serving Christ in all I do

For years I prayed for 'balance' in my work and never achieved it. One of my friends showed me a video where a CEO being interviewed told that if an airplane is going to crash they give the pre-flight instructions for you to put on your oxygen mask before you put on your child's.

The emphasis of this example is to take care of yourself before you try to help others. So for my 'oxygen' I starting saying I'd go to the YMCA and do an aerobic workout for 20 minutes/day and at least 42 sit-ups and 42 pushups a day. Soon the time grew and I began maximizing and optimizing my time to a minimum of 2 hours per day with aerobic, strength, and relaxation.

What is the oxygen mask you need to put on first daily?

_____

_____

_____

_____

What help could you be giving others that may actually be hurting them?

_____

_____

_____

_____

Here was an approximate schedule during that week: *Now as you read this remember this is after almost two years of following the Christian Revival Diet™ and my energy level has substantially increased. If I would have tried this schedule the first week, month or even within the first year, I would have burned myself out. So go gradually and most of all be good to yourself.

5:00 a.m.: wake and leave for work
(Workout clothes were already in the car on a hanger from the night before. Lunch was already made and in a bag ready to go next to a protein shake that will be drank post workout. The less I had to think about what I had to do in the morning the faster I could get out the door.)

5:05 a.m.: leave
(As I drive listen to a sermon on parenting. When I first got my current job I had a 25 minute commute, and I was so pent up and frustrated as I never had more than a 5 minute commute in my life. As a friend, Jon, introduced a radio station, locally KKMS 980AM, to me, where every half-hour they have a sermon. Soon after listening to various radio ministries I would plan my commute to leave on the hour or the ½ hour to catch a specific show. Now the smart phone can play these sermons on demand, I still listen to some of the broadcast via radio versions when they are available, otherwise I'll listen to the specific show on my way in.)

It changed my life!

Praise God! Actually it's still changing my life daily! Hallelujah!

5:35 a.m. arrive @ the YMCA

5:42 a.m.
(Swim 1st lap in the pool, finish my mile (between 72 and 88 lengths depending on the pool length) while meditating on God's word, my day, and where I can grow in my life.)

6:32 a.m.
(Exit the pool, say thanks to lifeguard, enter sauna, and edit pages of this book, jot down some fresh thoughts and notes)

7:00 a.m.
(Grab a mat and head to the boot camp class. Dru, the instructor and physical trainer, brings us through rigorous full body workout for 55 minutes)

8:00 a.m.
(Back to the sauna to rest, recover, perhaps read this manuscript or a newspaper, shave, shower, and dress)

8:15 a.m.
(Arrive at grocery store with the list my wife texted me. To shop when no one is there = just fresh vegetables this week)

8:30 a.m.
(Arrive @ work, drop two bags of groceries in the work refrigerator in the basement)

9:00 a.m.
(Work begins computer is up, daily duties are in line, emails are reviewed and deleted = working hard with intermittent breaks every 55 minutes to stretch, grab some water, and perhaps some pushups or crunches, or to brush my teeth)

12:30 p.m.
(Lunch is nibbled and then a quick 5k listening to a sermon on my smartphone followed with a shower @ work or @ the local YMCA 2 miles away)

1:30 p.m.
(Back to work and fresh, like it's a new day)

5:30 p.m.
(Shut down computer, review day and week calendar and clean desk for preparation for tomorrow)

6:15 p.m.

(On my commute, make a few phone calls or memorize a Bible verse. Then arrive @ home for dinner, family fun, kid's activities, clean up, devotions, reading, laundry, other household chores, etc.)

8:15 p.m.

(Children are tucked into bed, and now I'm off to writing, reading or relaxing)

9:00 p.m.

(A quick 10 minute yoga session is done by watching a good night time video on the internet, perhaps mute the words and choose a Bible verse to meditate on while watching or have a song in the background)

9:15 p.m.

(Quick review of my day, organize items, lunches, clothes, shakes, studies and priorities for the next day, review the Bible verse or listen to a sermon while doing the chores)

10:00 p.m.

(Lights out to pray and dream)

Guess what for me was the hardest part of this day?

You got it! Going to bed and turning the lights out, turning off the digital devices, and getting good sleep. The temptation for me was to get on the *wild goose-gle goose chase* searching for some articles on the stock markets, healthy living, politics, religion, or other thing on the internet.

The hardest challenge is limiting yourself and focusing. The realization that you can't do it all, and you have to focus on your part is vital.

In college I did the exercise for the model day as well and extended it out to the model week as the days were more varied.

It included the same type of things as above. My work was study time or campus jobs, and life without children just afforded more time for some of the other items and flexibility. What would your ideal daily or weekly schedule be:

_____

_____

_____

_____

_____

_____

_____

_____

_____

_____

_____

_____

_____

_____

_____

_____

_____

_____

_____

_____

_____

What is the most challenging part of the day for you to maintain and follow through on?

_____

_____

_____

_____

What prayer can you ask God to help you achieve focus in your improvement area of life?

_____

_____

_____

_____

Perform another short body/mind/soul scan and jot down what you are experiencing as a whole:

_____

_____

_____

_____

Please jot down any memories or thoughts that you need to let go of, forgive yourself or others, or confess and give to God in order to move forward with more health:

_____

_____

_____

How can you apply this to your life today in order be healthier:

_____

_____

_____

_____

"He who works with his hands is a laborer.
He who works with his hands and his head is a craftsman.
He who works with his hands, his head and his heart is an artist."

St. Francis of Assisi

How are you living a simple life focusing on what God wants you to?

_____

_____

_____

Living a quiet simple life today is harder than ever.

What is there to remember if you don't live fully?

_____

_____

_____

What is there to remember if you don't risk?

_____

_____

_____

What is there to remember if you don't love?

_____

_____

_____

8
REDEMPTION

"For all have sinned and fall short of the glory of God"
Romans 3:23

"For we are to God the pleasing aroma of Christ among those who are being saved and those who are perishing."

2 Corinthians 2:15

Redemption means an act of deliverance, rescue, forgiveness, or paying off debt.

Does your heart cry out to be redeemed?
If so, from what?
For what?
What sin?

Exodus 20 1:17

"And God spoke all these words:

I am the Lord your God, who brought you out of Egypt, out of the land of slavery.

You shall have no other gods before me.

You shall not make for yourself an idol in the form of anything in heaven above or on the earth beneath or in the waters below. You shall not bow down to them or worship them; for I, the Lord your God, am a jealous God, punishing the children for the sin of the fathers to the third and fourth generation of those who hate me, but showing love to a thousand generations of those who love me and keep my commandments.

You shall not misuse the name of the Lord your God, for the Lord will not hold anyone guiltless who misuses his name.

Remember the Sabbath day by keeping it holy. Six days you shall labor and do all your work, but the seventh day is a Sabbath to the Lord your God. On it you shall not do any work, neither you, nor your manservant or maidservant, nor your animals, nor the alien within your gates. For in six days the Lord made the heavens and the earth, the sea, and all that is in them, but he rested on the seventh day. Therefor the Lord blessed the Sabbath day and made it holy.

Honor your father and your mother, so that you may live long in the land the Lord your God is giving you.

You shall not murder.

You shall not commit adultery.

You shall not steal.

You shall not give false testimony against your neighbor.

You shall not covey your neighbor's house. You shall not covet your neighbor's wife, or his manservant or maidservant, his ox or donkey, or anything that belongs to your neighbor."

How do you compare your actions to the Ten Commandments?

_____

_____

_____

_____

How many times have you broken God's Ten Commandments? How many sins do you need to be redeemed from if each were put on trial?

_____

_____

_____

How many sins have you committed?

_____

_____

Imagine all your thoughts, deeds… Isn't it amazing how we self-rationalize our behavior typically in terms of others to justify our current appropriateness or sin? Often saying, I'm better than them or I'm better more of the time, or I'm not as bad as the other person.

I can't even count that high or that far.

Thank God for grace! Words can't explain the thankfulness.

Thank God for redemption that Jesus paid it all for our grace, once and for all finished.

I love you Jesus!

Now that you are redeemed what is the greatest calling for you to do?

It's to serve Christ.

To become self-forgetful, but not self-neglectful. In order to serve God you need to honor your body. As Holy Spirit resides in you, you can be the most effective for God by taking care of yourself. Refresh by re-reading 1 Corinthians 6:19-20

Could you be strengthening your health to serve Christ better? In what areas?

_____

_____

_____

Humility comes from the Latin word "humus" which means soil. Human comes from that word as well. Isn't it interesting that from dust we came and from dust we return. Due to modern science and the study of the elements, we are just matter that will return to the matter that is all part of the soil. We are comprised of these items: oxygen, carbon, hydrogen, nitrogen, calcium, phosphorus, potassium, sulfur, sodium, magnesium, copper, zinc, selenium, molybdenum, fluorine, chlorine, iodine, manganese, cobalt, iron, lithium, strontium, aluminum, silicon, lead, vanadium, arsenic, bromine.

Genesis 2:7
"Then the Lord God formed a man from the dust of the ground and breathed into his nostrils the breath of life, and the man became a living being."

5000+ years later, it's conclusive we are relatively boring from a pure particle make up. With the particle make up, common dirt would seem more expansive than our boring 28 particles. But the thousands of combinations that come together make our vital organs, matter, neurons that the only explanation that God.

God even said in Genesis 3:19:

"By the sweat of your brow you will eat your food until you return to the ground, since from it you were taken; for dust you are and to dust you

will return."

So, during the time when your earthly particles (dust) were first put together to the time they return to dust, may you uncover the meaning of what you were put here to do:

What do you think you were put here to do?

_____

_____

_____

_____

God spoke about that as well in Isaiah 43:7 *"whom I created for my glory"*

Indeed, in 1 Corinthians 10:31 it's highlighted, *"So whether you eat or drink or whatever you do, do it all for the glory of God."*

What does doing everything for God's glory look like in your life?

_____

_____

God is in control and totally sovereign. He does not need one thing from us. However, the purpose he made us for was to glorify and bring glory to Him in all we do and tell others about Him.

God is sovereign, meaning that He is completely independent. He did not need to create us. He does not need us for anything. Based on this we might come to the conclusion that we are not important to God.... that we are not needed and we have no purpose. But, that's not the end of the story. God tells us in Scripture that we were created to glorify Him. That's our purpose and that means we are important to Him personally.

We glorify God by:

Trusting His promises

Our desire to obey Him

Our desire to know Him

Our desire is to love Him with our body, mind and soul

So read Galatians 5:1
"It is for freedom that Christ has set us free. Stand firm, then, and do not let yourselves be burdened again by a yoke of slavery."

What does it mean to you? What are you in slavery to?

_____

_____

_____

How can you apply it to your life?

_____

_____

Reality strikes hard though. Although we know the message and know the story of our Redeemer, we too often build our life on other things.

How do you base your decisions?

Peers
Pros
Cons
Economics
Fact
Feelings
Emotions
World
Church
Pastor

Friend
Family
Co-worker
Logic
Cross of Jesus
Call
Faith
Testing what is true

Have you had a crossroads moment where you have had to choose what you think God is telling you to do and someone else is challenging you to do? How did you make your decision?

_____

_____

_____

Personally, the church I had attended for 13 years didn't take a proactive stand on a recent issue that affected our state at an election. There was limited guidance and no real discernment for direction or clarity.

The hard truth was that my wife and I had to make a decision, either we leave that church based on this situation and the set of circumstances facing us or stay and tolerate the weak leadership on these pertinent issues, where the Bible was in clear conflict with the teaching of the church (or lack of teaching).

I used to think that it was my fault for not speaking up, and I still do to a certain extent. But then my thoughts tried to blame the government for allowing some of these blatant and now acceptable sins that permeate our schools, churches, institutions of leadership and our businesses.

What I now realize is that looking at desire for global revival the scapegoating is often to the above areas, but frankly it's a failure of leadership from the pulpit and my own ignorant laziness in not reading and acting upon the Bible as God was breathing it into me.

We, the sheep, have been led astray by wimpy pastors not willing to take the stand for truth, God's word, and the call of their leadership. They've opted for tolerance to fill the seats and trying to "woo" the parishioners giving them subtle messages with a "velvet hammer".....strike that, more like a "velvet marshmallow" sweet, addictive and seemingly without any immediate consequence. However in the long run there will be consequences.

Jesus Christ is always good and always loves you, your church. He is 100% in control. So He knows what He is doing. At first I questioned why He was allowing the church to get soft. But one of my applications through this is that the counterfeits are more easily identifiable. So I had to discern if this going to be a place to continue to support and participate in if the message wasn't consistent with my understanding of God's will.

Clarity brings the strong answer "No way". Time to move on. (We did confront, however, by working with more than a half-dozen other parishioners and speaking to four senior pastors and only receiving even weaker responses).

This begets the question, where do you get your opinions and put your trust? These areas have to be discerned and held to God's lens. There is no perfect church and I understand that. Once I think I've found the perfect church, I better not go there, as I will ruin it.

However, there are better churches. May God guide you in the direction you need to go. And that your eyes will not be blind to the realities of Biblically solid doctrine that your church should stand on.

In another practical example, here is a letter I sent to my son's hockey coaches as the kids were rough housing a bit, and we needed to unify leadership.
"Dear Coaches (please forward if you have the core coaches' email or any of the other coaches),

This is an observation, potential solution, I send it through seeking your feedback, approval or to solicit other ideas.

I spoke with *the core coach* post practice and he is 100% on board. I'll draft the talking points that would be good to emphasize and set expectations to. I was fortunate to go to an awesome soccer practice later in the day today where the coach laid out his expectations. So for the next 44+ sessions of practice and learning, I'd suggest we get unified along some lines. If we are 70% in agreement on these, let's encourage adherence to 100% along these lines.

This is what I was thinking about communicating with encouragement and follow through to the kids. (Any ideas, suggestions, amendments... it's better to set the tone at the beginning of the year.)

1) We are here first and foremost to be safe, do what the coaches say, and that is how we have fun playing hockey. Fun is not the most important thing nor is winning. Safety and doing what you are told is what is the most important. You have fun by doing this, and we, as your coaches, have fun too. Whether you win or lose, the lessons you learn to grow through this are the most vital. So smile and let's have fun by listening with our eyes and ears open, your mouth closed and being safe out here.

2) You listen with your eyes and ears open and your mouths closed. When any of the coaches speak you give them 100% attention that means looking at them (not the guy sitting next to you, or not the crowd). We know it's hard to hear on the ice, but it's harder to hear when you are looking away, have your back to us or aren't listening, and you are talking. This will not be allowed on our team.

3) You are here to play and learn and have fun so give it your 100% by doing the drills you are requested to do the best you can. You can improve, but you must do the drills like we tell you.

You will be sent to your parents and not able to play or put in the penalty box, for if you breach any of the following items. As if you are doing any of the following things, it is a message to us that you really don't want to play hockey on our team.

a) If you are horse playing around, pushing, shoving, hitting, tripping, negative or discouraging words to other players, putting your stick in other peoples skates, not listening with your eyes or listening with your ears to your coaches, interrupting your coaches.

b) No crashing into your team when you exit the ice on a drill. You'll get a chance to play, it's not a race, be gracious and fair. Don't push, shove or trip, we want quality play.

c) If the coach calls "LINE CHECK" you must look at the coach, stand at attention and hold your stick with both hands directly holding the stick. Let's have fun by listening with our eyes, respecting and encouraging each other, while doing our best. You are great kids with lots of potential let's achieve success.
Can we do this?!?!? (Ideally teams cheers! yeah! yeah! =
Respect, listening and doing your best

Commentary:
This is the message I heard today while at our soccer practice, but summarized from our hockey team's perspective. It has been communicated now 3 weeks to the soccer team we are on, and the kids' are getting it. I know the youth hockey players need to hear this message.

The only way I'd communicate this is if we are going to stand behind and enforce it. Gentleman, I don't have any of the other team's coach's emails, but I think they'd grow as well from this message. I'm happy to communicate it, but we all need to keep this in front of the kids to create consistency and ideally just create it as "how" we do things on our team, as well if the other teams buy into it.

The core coach mentioned he is 100% on board.

If these are our expectations, let's tell the kids and enforce our expectations. They want our leadership and they are eager to comply.

Please send through any thoughts, your concurrence or another solution? And forward to any of the other coaches if you have their emails and approve of this message.

BTW I'm out next weekend for both practices/games. But we could do this Sunday am, if you get this and approve of it. The challenge is that it takes 3-4 times to reinforce at this age level to garner their trust, consistency and followership typically.

Thanks

DE"

The amazing thing with the communication above is that 7-8 parent coaches all received the message. They all commented to me 1-1 that the message was the right thing to deliver, but no one wanted to stand and say it. More than half commented that they didn't want to be labeled as the 'bad' guy.

So when did doing what is right and enforcing the rules devolve into being the bad guy? Or the bad dad?

No historical monologue here today about how the media helped portray truth and righteous living as bad, it just seems that we keep repeating the past without regard for the future.

We need faith and yet we need action. The challenge is that we've been paralyzed by trying to appeal to the negativity and keep letting the inmates run the crumbling asylums. Those who oppose the righteous and virtuous things win over in the short term, but our lack of confidence and our ability to stand firm is where we are to blame. The faith we have can only come from God @ the center.

Imagine what happens to a culture and a people who aren't ever given clear direction or the proper path.
Are you desperate for change? Are you desperate to communicate truth?

_____

_____

_____

_____

"For God so loved the world that he gave his one and only Son, that whoever believes in him shall not perish but have eternal life. For God did not send his Son into the world to condemn the world, but to save the world through him."

John 3:16-3:17

"Our Father in heaven,
Hallowed be your name,
Your kingdom come,
Your will be done,
On earth as it is in Heaven.

Give us this day our daily bread.
And forgive us our debts,
As we also have forgiven our debtors.
And lead us not into temptation,
But deliver us from the evil one."

Matthew 6:9-13

These are some of the most quoted Bible verses, but they need to be fully digested to see the fruit. Like so many times some of the greatest things we become familiar with, are too often the things that lose their potency based on our familiarity. The unthinking rote recitation is dangerous when it comes to these things. So, hopefully, these questions can get you thinking and, most importantly, applying some of these truths to your life.

Why did God send His son to die for you?

_____

_____

_____

Why didn't God send His son to die for you?

_____

_____

_____

Whose will do we pray will get done?

_____

_____

_____

What are key and essential that we need to do today?

_____

_____

_____

Who do we need to forgive?

_____

_____

_____

Where should we be led and delivered from?

_____

_____

_____

All of the answers should show the inherent need for a spiritual revival in your life. The Christian Revival Diet™ has told you this again.

How are you putting food, drink, entertainment, or lusts of the flesh above Christ?

_____

_____

_____

What goal are you working on now?

_____

_____

_____

How desperate are you for the goal?

_____

_____

_____

I am not here to judge and I can't judge.

Only God can judge!

I can assess and make a personal bias on my level of engagement on what someone else is doing, whether to participate or to turn away. That is as far as I can go regarding my discernment and involvement. But I am not able to judge.

Everyone will give an account. What would the summary of your account sound like?

_____

_____

_____

Is there anything in your life that you won't let go?

_____

_____

_____

What is standing in the way of Christ fully getting in?

_____

_____

_____

What trials are you facing?

_____

_____

_____

Would Christ be honored by the following as He is watching all aspects of our lives?

...the music we listen to...
...the drink we drink...
...the food we eat...
...the church we attend...
...the jokes we tell...
...our intentional ambition...
...the words that come from our mouth...
...the sins we tolerate...
...the books we read or write...
...the people we spend our time with...
...what resources we hold onto for us...

Circle those above that Christ would be pleased with

Add extra below:

_____

_____

_____

_____

_____

_____

_____

It's not about being legalistic, it's about truth.

Remember that song:

Be careful little eyes what you see...

Some of the other verses include....

Be careful little mouth what you say....
Be careful little ears what you hear....
Be careful little hands what you do....
Be careful little feet where you go...

There is a Father up above
Looking down with tender love
So, be careful little mouth what you say,
> hear, do, say, and where you go.

The song was written during a difficult time. We have always lived in tumultuous times. Since we got booted out of the Garden of Eden we've had some tough times and death has been part of our reality. Sad, but true. Once you realize this the surprise of the challenges and pains in the world should not keep surprise you any longer.

Isn't it funny how during times of peace people make problems for themselves and during times of challenge people strive and make improvements?

God can see all of time at the same time. He is truly limitless and knows everything. Imagine if you had no sense of time. The only reality was eternity, and you could see everything happening at once.

When asked how to live the Christian life, here are some of the typical responses you might hear:

Church attendance
Bible study
Prayer
Memory verses
Fellowship
Confession
Religion
Daily quiet time

Singing songs
Meditation
Worship

It's interesting to consider these are all rituals, and a true Christian life stems from the heart. It should permeate everything you do.

The list contains all good things to do, but at the end of the there is only one thing that is living the Christian life and that is Christ. Christ is the Christian life, on everything else this hangs.

It's not about you.....

Are you wallowing, whining, or wandering in the wilderness?

How do you make your decisions?

Peer pressure
Pros/cons
Opinions
Fact
Emotions
Feelings
World
Financial
Logic
Avoidance
Jesus Christ is always good and always loves you, so how should you make decisions?

Christ's silence is not a sign of absence. Perhaps it's requiring you to grow stronger through this trial. Perhaps it's challenging you to take a greater leadership role and take a stand.

The side affects you may see are perspiration, desperation, and that only comes from a demonstration of faith.

So how is your perspiration, desperation and demonstration of faith being shown to others?

_____

_____

_____

There is only one place to put your hope in, and that is Jesus Christ.

Maturity is the ability to defer pleasure.

9

RESURRECTION

"Jesus turned and said to them, 'Daughters of Jerusalem, do not weep for me; weep for yourselves and for your children. For the time will come when you will say, 'Blessed are the childless women, the wombs that never bore and the breasts that never nursed!' Then 'they will say to the mountains, 'Fall on us!' and to the hills, 'Cover us!'''

For if people do these things when the tree is green, what will happen when it is dry?"

Two other men, both criminals, were also led out with him to be executed. When they came to the place called the Skull, they crucified him there, along with the criminals—one on his right, the other on his left. Jesus said, "Father, forgive them, for they do not know what they are doing." And they divided up his clothes by casting lots."

Luke 23:28-32

I repeat: *"weep for yourselves and for your children. For the time will come when you will say, 'Blessed are the childless women, the wombs that never bore and the breasts that never nursed!"*

Dreadful. Nevertheless, it's a stern wake up call.

For Jesus to say for us to weep for yourselves and later to say that blessed are the childless women seems a bit extreme.

Is this even comprehendible that this type of attitude could prevail in our modern, technological advanced, and savvy world?

The reality is that at any given time on this earth there is someone saying that they don't want to bring a child into the world due to war, selfish goals, or economic fears. The sad reality is that this is reflected often in our society.

Our society has shied away from hearing about sin or dealing with sin directly. Shied away from the tough message.

As some young married couples question having children fearful of bringing them into this world with some of the issues.

From Luke 23:34 *"Jesus said, "Father, forgive them, for they do not know what they are doing."*

In order to know what resurrection is you must know where you are coming from. Jesus was resurrected. He was reborn out of physical death brought back to eternal life. That is what will happen to us if we accept Him in our life. Only He has the power to save us. In order be reborn and resurrected out of our sins, we must die to ourselves. Ourselves being our sinful nature.

My turning point and conversion moment was when I was at church standing at a service listening to a song. As I closed my eyes my mind went someplace I wasn't expecting.

I was suddenly on a razor sharp mountain peak, actually more of a needle point without any sides. Everywhere I looked

I saw only darkness. Down all sides was the depth of eternity, falling without a net, or anything to catch me. I was standing there alone and the fear of falling was gripping me.

It seemed like an eternity there, but it must have been only a few moments as when I opened my eyes the song was still playing.

I realized at that moment the depth of my depravity and the conviction of my sin. I realized life without God and what the eternal Abyss was. About 5 years later I was reading Revelation 9:1-12 where it speaks about the Abyss. Before that time I had never heard a sermon about that, nor did I ever read that passage, or if I read it I never really heard it. I didn't want to really focus on that harsh truth.

The image of it, and the feeling of emptiness and bitterness, overwhelms my soul to the point of pain and tears every time I remember that feeling.

Looking back, I wish that early on someone had spoken the hard and honest truth to me. I'm sure they did but I didn't listen. I wanted to do it my way. And boy I did…. Fortunately, the turning point sent me on a path to dig deeper in Christ and really develop a relationship with Him as well.

Have you had a conversion moment? What was it?

_____

_____

_____

_____

What do you wish someone had warned you about earlier?

_____

_____

_____

_____

What can you warn others about when you see them stray?

_____

_____

_____

_____

_____

Amazingly enough, in order to know righteousness, sadly, you have to point out what is unrighteous and what is indeed sin, and be convicted of it to the point where you want to run away from the sin and stop doing what you are doing.

The greatest challenge in our day is that many pastors, preachers, lay people, and parents don't want to point out the reality of sin, and thus we have unconvinced, unconverted, and un-convicted Christians more amused by the religion and rituals of Christianity than a true change of heart. Just like counterfeit foods we have counterfeit Christians.

The heart must change; otherwise you will find yourself back at the same point or worse. The resurrection gives you the depth behind the drive to achieve. You must die to yourself and live in Christ.

Sin means separation or transgression or missing the mark, and we all are separated, falling short, missing the mark and transgressing.

Some sin more than others.

Sin is sin.

Some of the sins our world likes to highlight are some of the core things that we may look down on are and even have laws around as well:

Murder

Lying

Stealing

Cheating

Infidelity

But let's go a little deeper into
the reality of what God calls sin.

Idol worship

Pride

Jealousy

Lust of the eyes

Sexual immorality

Greed

Slander

Wanting something that is not yours

The Ten Commandments are the law and the frame to hold everything up to. So we can look at what to strive not to do by studying them. Here is another verse to learn about what not to do, and what God calls sin.

Deuteronomy 27:15-26 highlights where people will be cursed:

The Levites shall recite to all the people of Israel in a loud voice:

[15] *"Cursed is anyone who makes an idol—a thing detestable to the LORD, the work of skilled hands—and sets it up in secret."*

Then all the people shall say, "Amen!"

¹⁶ *"Cursed is anyone who dishonors their father or mother."*

Then all the people shall say, "Amen!"

¹⁷ *"Cursed is anyone who moves their neighbor's boundary stone."*

Then all the people shall say, "Amen!"

¹⁸ *"Cursed is anyone who leads the blind astray on the road."*

Then all the people shall say, "Amen!"

¹⁹ *"Cursed is anyone who withholds justice from the foreigner, the fatherless or the widow."*

Then all the people shall say, "Amen!"

²⁰ *"Cursed is anyone who sleeps with his father's wife, for he dishonors his father's bed."*

Then all the people shall say, "Amen!"

²¹ *"Cursed is anyone who has sexual relations with any animal."*

Then all the people shall say, "Amen!"

²² *"Cursed is anyone who sleeps with his sister, the daughter of his father or the daughter of his mother."*

Then all the people shall say, "Amen!"

²³ *"Cursed is anyone who sleeps with his mother-in-law."*

Then all the people shall say, "Amen!"

²⁴ *"Cursed is anyone who kills their neighbor secretly."*

Then all the people shall say, "Amen!"

25 "Cursed is anyone who accepts a bribe to kill an innocent person."

Then all the people shall say, "Amen!"

26 "Cursed is anyone who does not uphold the words of this law by carrying them out."

Then all the people shall say, "Amen!"

While some might say that since it's from the Old Testament some things have changed. Well, then, let's look closer at the New Testament as well. Galatians 5:16-26

16 So I say, walk by the Spirit, and you will not gratify the desires of the flesh. 17 For the flesh desires what is contrary to the Spirit, and the Spirit what is contrary to the flesh. They are in conflict with each other, so that you are not to do whatever[c] you want. 18 But if you are led by the Spirit, you are not under the law.

19 The acts of the flesh are obvious: sexual immorality, impurity and debauchery; 20 idolatry and witchcraft; hatred, discord, jealousy, fits of rage, selfish ambition, dissensions, factions 21 and envy; drunkenness, orgies, and the like. I warn you, as I did before, that those who live like this will not inherit the kingdom of God.

22 But the fruit of the Spirit is love, joy, peace, forbearance, kindness, goodness, faithfulness, 23 gentleness and self-control. Against such things there is no law. 24 Those who belong to Christ Jesus have crucified the flesh with its passions and desires. 25 Since we live by the Spirit, let us keep in step with the Spirit. 26 Let us not become conceited, provoking and envying each other."

Wow! Have you heard your pastor preaching about this recently? Without preaching about it, how can revival occur?

Your life will only change to the level of truth that you proclaim or hear.

The truth that you proclaim rises to the level of Christ's claim on you.

He claimed you. How will you comply?

———————————————————————

———————————————————————

One of the Biblical verses that highlight His claim on you:

"Do you not know that your bodies are temples of the Holy Spirit, who is in you, whom you have received from God? You are not your own; you were bought at a price. Therefore honor God with your bodies."
1 Corinthians 6:19-20

"For we are God's handiwork, created in Christ Jesus to do good works, which God prepared in advance for us to do."
Ephesians 2:10

Indeed the greatest challenge to some of these more subtle sins is that God doesn't separate and value sins differently. Like in the Matthew verses about looking lustfully at a woman is like committing the sin. Like being angry at a brother is like murder them. These are tough teachings and ever so challenging to apply to our daily lives.

Integration, however is key. God is patient, slow to anger and loving. He cares for you and wants your full obedience. At this point he doesn't demand it. He allows you to do your dance, but he weeps for you with open arms calling you back to Him every step of your day.

What, then, are the boundaries and standards God has set for us that define sin? The most basic definition of sin is in the Ten Commandments and keys to the Christian Revival Diet™. If you live like this, you will surely find peace. The peace that surpasses all understanding. Hold up God's law:

Exodus 20:

And God spoke all these words:

"I am the LORD *your God, who brought you out of Egypt, out of the land of slavery.*

"You shall have no other gods before[a] me.

"You shall not make for yourself an image in the form of anything in heaven above or on the earth beneath or in the waters below. ⁵ You shall not bow down to them or worship them; for I, the LORD *your God, am a jealous God, punishing the children for the sin of the parents to the third and fourth generation of those who hate me, ⁶ but showing love to a thousand generations of those who love me and keep my commandments.*

"You shall not misuse the name of the LORD *your God, for the* LORD *will not hold anyone guiltless who misuses his name.*

"Remember the Sabbath day by keeping it holy. ⁹ Six days you shall labor and do all your work, ¹⁰ but the seventh day is a Sabbath to the LORD *your God. On it you shall not do any work, neither you, nor your son or daughter, nor your male or female servant, nor your animals, nor any foreigner residing in your towns. ¹¹ For in six days the* LORD *made the heavens and the earth, the sea, and all that is in them, but he rested on the seventh day. Therefore the* LORD *blessed the Sabbath day and made it holy.*

"Honor your father and your mother, so that you may live long in the land the LORD *your God is giving you.*

"You shall not murder.

"You shall not commit adultery.

"You shall not steal.

"You shall not give false testimony against your neighbor.

"You shall not covet your neighbor's house. You shall not covet your neighbor's wife, or his male or female servant, his ox or donkey, or anything that belongs to your neighbor."

When the people saw the thunder and lightning and heard the trumpet and saw the mountain in smoke, they trembled with fear. They stayed at a distance and said to Moses, "Speak to us yourself and we will listen. But do not have God speak to us or we will die."

At a Big Ten football game today, 78,000 people enjoyed three or so hours of screaming, cheering, and shouting while eating large bratwursts and drinking beer. It was a great game. The talent did wonderfully on the field, and the crowd participated with the enthusiasm typical of a college crowd.

TV can draw crowds of 20 million people sitting on couches gazing at 200-700 channels and seemingly unlimited internet resources to search. The challenge lies in discerning what is most important to view and spend our time on.

The Department of Labor did an analysis of where Americans spent their time in 2012 per day.

Sleeping	= 8:44 hours/day
Work-related activities	= 3:32 hours/day
Watching television	= 2:50 hours/day
Leisure and sports	= 2:32 hours/day
Household activities	= 1:44 hours/day
Eating and drinking	= 1:15 hours/day
Personal Care	= 0:45 hours/day
Shopping	= 0:44 hours/day

The other 2-3 hours per day is spent caring for other people, civic and religious activities, email, etc.

I've read commentaries where people estimate that the Neanderthal man had to work hard 20 hours per week if living in a warm climate to sustain shelter, food and lack of clothing. No one really knows, but now with the 24 hour society and electricity powering everything our ability to do more and produce more has grown with the complexity of longer work weeks, different kinds of stressors and such.

If the average person lives to be 80 years old with 365 days per year, that'd be 29,200 days. In 29,200 days that'd mean 700,800 hours. However with 1/3 of the hours on sleeping, hygiene or eating that lower it to under 470,000 hours to apply your gifts to the world around you. Deduct the formative years (13-26) with education and learning and the later years that are filled with reduced application and cognitive function (80+), and there is truly not much time to apply your learning. Some might have 30 years or 10952 days give or take a few.

The challenge is that it goes by so quickly, so the point is to invest your time wisely, with people and things that are going are the most important. How much are you fully in control of what you are viewing, doing, or engaging in?

Sin is everywhere. Let's continue learning about what the Bible says about sin and what is does in our life.

1 John 3:4 *"Everyone who sins breaks the law; in fact, sin is lawlessness."*

Everyone sins, so we are all lawless.

"See, I set before you today life and prosperity, death and destruction. [16] For I command you today to love the LORD your God, to walk in obedience to him, and to keep his commands, decrees and laws; then you will live and increase, and the LORD your God will bless you in the land you are entering to possess."

Deuteronomy 30:15-16

When we sin we violate the law of love.

Matthew 15:17-20

"Don't you see that whatever enters the mouth goes into the stomach and then out of the body? But the things that come out of a person's mouth come from the heart, and these defile them. For out of the heart come evil thoughts—murder, adultery, sexual immorality, theft, false testimony, slander. These are what defile a person; but eating with unwashed hands does not defile them."

From a worldly perspective, we often don't see much wrong with allowing unrighteous thoughts into our minds. The thoughts are sometimes quite pleasurable and entertaining. However eventually these sinful thoughts will lead us into greater temptation which can lead to deeper sin. The result is the trampling of God's law. Jesus Christ instructs us to disrupt that process before it gets started, by not even allowing wrong thoughts into our minds.

From Romans 14

"Accept the one whose faith is weak, without quarreling over disputable matters. One person's faith allows them to eat anything, but another, whose faith is weak, eats only vegetables. The one who eats everything must not treat with contempt the one who does not, and the one who does not eat everything must not judge the one who does, for God has accepted them. Who are you to judge someone else's servant? To their own master, servants stand or fall. And they will stand, for the Lord is able to make them stand.

One person considers one day more sacred than another; another considers every day alike. Each of them should be fully convinced in their own mind. Whoever regards one day as special does so to the Lord. Whoever eats meat does so to the Lord, for they give thanks to God; and whoever abstains does so to the Lord and gives thanks to God. For none of us lives for ourselves alone, and none of us dies for ourselves alone. If we live, we live for the Lord; and if we die, we die for the Lord. So, whether we live or die, we belong to the Lord. [9] For this very reason, Christ died and returned to life so that he might be the Lord of both the dead and the living.

You, then, why do you judge your brother or sister? Or why do you treat them with contempt? For we will all stand before God's judgment seat. It is written:

*"'As surely as I live,' says the Lord,
'every knee will bow before me;
every tongue will acknowledge God.'"*

So then, each of us will give an account of ourselves to God.

Therefore let us stop passing judgment on one another. Instead, make up your mind not to put any stumbling block or obstacle in the way of a brother or sister. I am convinced, being fully persuaded in the Lord Jesus, that nothing is unclean in itself. But if anyone regards something as unclean, then for that person it is unclean. If your brother or sister is distressed because of what you eat, you are no longer acting in love. Do not by your eating destroy someone for whom Christ died. Therefore do not let what you know is good be spoken of as evil. For the kingdom of God is not a matter of eating and drinking, but of righteousness, peace and joy in the Holy Spirit, because anyone who serves Christ in this way is pleasing to God and receives human approval.

Let us therefore make every effort to do what leads to peace and to mutual edification. [20] Do not destroy the work of God for the sake of food. All food is clean, but it is wrong for a person to eat anything that causes someone else to stumble. It is better not to eat meat or drink wine or to do anything else that will cause your brother or sister to fall.

So whatever you believe about these things keep between yourself and God. Blessed is the one who does not condemn himself by what he approves. But whoever has doubts is condemned if they eat, because their eating is not from faith; and everything that does not come from faith is sin."

What application do you see that comes from Romans 14?

_____

_____

_____

_____

The Gospels are filled with many examples of sin. Christ often called the religious people of His day, "blind guides", "brood of vipers", and "hypocrites". These religious people searched to follow Biblical teaching by following strict obedience of God's law, and failed to realize that God expected the greater sacrifice of grace and love in comparison to following the strict ideals. The Pharisees wasted a bunch of emotional energy trying to confront Jesus about healing people on the Sabbath. Instead of rejoicing in His healing, they tried to hold Him accountable for his breaking the work rule.

In fact, they wanted to kill Christ. Now you see why Christ called them some of those nasty names.

Matthew 25:31-46

"When the Son of Man comes in his glory, and all the angels with him, he will sit on his glorious throne. All the nations will be gathered before him, and he will separate the people one from another as a shepherd separates the sheep from the goats. He will put the sheep on his right and the goats on his left.

Then the King will say to those on the right, 'Come, you who are blessed by my Father take your inheritance, the kingdom prepared for you since the creation of the world. For I was hungry and you gave me something to eat, I was thirsty and you gave me something to drink, I was a stranger and you invited me in, I needed clothes and you clothed me, I was sick and you looked after me, I was in prison and you came to visit me.

Then the righteous will answer him, 'Lord, when did we see you hungry and feed you, or thirsty and give you something to drink? When did we see you a stranger and invite you in, or needing clothes and clothe you? When did we see you sick or in prison and go to visit you?

The King will reply, 'Truly I tell you, whatever you did for one of the least of these brothers and sisters of mine, you did for me.'

Then he will say to those on his left, 'Depart from me, you who are cursed, into the eternal fire prepared for the devil and his angels. For I was hungry and you gave me nothing to eat, I was thirsty and you gave me nothing to drink, ⁴³ I was a stranger and you did not invite me in, I needed clothes and you did not clothe me, I was sick and in prison and you did not look after me.'

"They also will answer, 'Lord, when did we see you hungry or thirsty or a stranger or needing clothes or sick or in prison, and did not help you?'

"He will reply, 'Truly I tell you, whatever you did not do for one of the least of these, you did not do for me.'

"Then they will go away to eternal punishment, but the righteous to eternal life."

Where in your life are you trying to right your sins with your actions?

_____

_____

_____

In James 2:14-24 it's highlighted:

"What good is it, my brothers and sisters, if someone claims to have faith but has no deeds? Can such faith save them? ¹⁵ Suppose a brother or a sister is without clothes and daily food. ¹⁶ If one of you says to them, "Go in peace; keep warm and well fed," but does nothing about their physical needs, what good is it? In the same way, faith by itself, if it is not accompanied by action, is dead.

But someone will say, "You have faith; I have deeds."

Show me your faith without deeds, and I will show you my faith by my deeds. You believe that there is one God. Good! Even the demons believe that—and shudder.

You foolish person, do you want evidence that faith without deeds is useless? Was not our father Abraham considered righteous for what he did when he offered his son Isaac on the altar? You see that his faith and his actions were working together, and his faith was made complete by what he did. And the scripture was fulfilled that says, "Abraham believed God, and it was credited to him as righteousness," and he was called God's friend. You see that a person is considered righteous by what they do and not by faith alone."

What is your takeaway from the James passage?

_____

_____

_____

What is your new call for action?

_____

_____

What are you doing to revive your mind?

_____

_____

What addictions, fears, pains, and maladies do you want out of your life?

_____

_____

_____

What do you crave?

_____

_____

_____

_____

What do you desire?

_____

_____

_____

What do you lack?

_____

_____

_____

10
REFRESH

"And the Lord's servant must not be quarrelsome but must be kind to everyone, able to teach, not resentful. Opponents must be gently instructed, in the hope that God will grant them repentance leading them to the knowledge of the truth, and that they will come to their senses and escape from the trap of the devil, who has taken them captive to do his will."

2 Timothy 2:24-26

The face of the surgeon.

The cry of a newborn baby.

The scurry of midwives, nurses and doctors moving rapidly to do their work after the birth of our youngest son Daniel. Anne, my wife complained that she was cold as they were toweling off Daniel and she was waiting to hold him. I was comforting her crouched next to the bed.

The birth had gone faster than expected. But for child #3, I guess my wife had been to this rodeo before. The laboring was less than an hour and within a few pushes the baby was out.

Anne again complained that she was cold.

I asked the nurse for a blanket or a towel, but a few towels later Anne still said she was cold. We were focused on the baby and Anne's cold, not the midwife who was cleaning up. Soon there was a very high stack of bloody towels accumulating on the rolling tray next to the midwife.

That is when I saw him.

The man with the eagle eye and the fox like face. Everyone else was smiling and doing their duties. He entered with eyes and an expression like I have never seen before. It was like a lion mother inspecting her cubs in a field of hyenas. He had eagle-like eyes and lightly browned skin that was tight around his jaw bone. His eyes surveyed everything, and he walked right up to Anne and asked how she was doing?

Anne said, "I am just so cold."

The man looked at me and I nervously said hello. His gaze went right through me as if summoned by a greater call. He told to me to take the baby from Anne and go over to the other side of the room. I complied, but as I looked backed at Anne her eyes screamed that something was wrong as she gasped and grasped to keep holding the baby.

I asked the nurse "what might be wrong?"

She said she didn't know.

"Who is that man by the table is talking with the mid-wife."

She said, "That is the surgeon."

Confused my mind raced wondering why a surgeon was here. This is our third child and Anne has been such a trooper. She never even had pain medication. She never had any doctors involved in the past, just midwives.

Quickly, the surgeon said to me we need to figure out a way to stop the bleeding.

I gasped "Well, will everything be ok?"

He replied, "We don't know but usually it is something we can take care of in 30 minutes to an hour, if all goes well."

As quickly as he said that, everyone left the room. All that was left was a table full of towels covered in blood and me holding my baby. I was stunned and shell-shocked.

About fifteen minutes went by before a nurse came by to clean and tidy up the room, when she said, "Oh, sorry, we forgot about you. Let me chat with the head nurse and see where you can wait during the surgery."

Soon I was put into an empty room with a couch at the far end facing the door which seemed at least fifty feet away. It had a tunnel like effect when looking at the door. The door opened and a nurse just stood there.

"How is she doing, and how long will she be in surgery?" I asked.

Graciously and empathetically, the nurse said, "We don't know. However, we think it will be another hour or so."

Two hours past as I sat on the couch holding my newborn, singing two songs: "Blessings" by Laura Story and "Come Thou Font of Every Blessing" over and over.

The nurse entered and the outline of her body was the

only thing I could see. The nurse just stood in the door and heard my singing as I gradually lowered the volume. Without saying anything she approached the distant doorway slowly.

I asked, "Is she ok?"

"We don't know." The nurse stuttered and came a couple steps closer, though still very shyly.

"Well, is she going to make it?" I asked sternly.

"The surgeon is doing his best. We don't know at this point, but I will keep you updated. She asked if I had any family near that could be with me."

You may wonder, why this is in the last chapter and how it relates to refresh? What has this to do encouraging healthy lifestyles?

Well I still see daily the surgeon's eyes and face when I am faced with tough leadership situations that I encounter which take extra focus and discernment to see to the core of what God really wants me to do.

The surgeon was coming into a life-threatening situation. There were no pleasantries, no talk about the weather, and generalities of entertainment where exchanged, just a goal of saving a life. His approach was necessary and determined.

In relating this to the Christian Revival Diet™ or otherwise a healthy revival in our land is to see our role like the surgeon sees his role.

The surgeon's laser-like focus centered on the problem and sought the solution using all his talent, knowledge, skills, and ability. Emotions were put on the shelf. At first I thought he was quite aloof and a bit unsympathetic, but looking back I see his aim was clear, his resolve was solid, and his focus totally on the problem. He showed true care by going to the source with the utmost diligence to serve the true need.

When it is life and death we definitely act fast. However the challenge is that we don't know when death will come. And we prefer to be liked or have people live in comfort of 'having it your way' or 'doing things as you like it' versus understanding the risks of the life and death scenarios that are in our midst.

So many scenarios, unlike the above, may not seem life and death. But knowing that Jesus' message, "Repent for the kingdom of heaven is near" shines the light of reality that the eternal consequences of life and death are real. These choices play out daily and actually played out for everyone everywhere.

In this scenario, if the surgeon hadn't had the focus, knowledge, determination, and obedience to his calling and craft, my wife may not have survived the 4 hours in surgery and the 5 days in the ICU. Praise God for those who have the true care for the focus on eternity, as so many have the counterfeit care and lack of evaluating the core issue. The issue is that this world is in need of a spiritual surgeon.

In every interaction, when confronted with challenging issues, sinful behavior, wrong choices, you can choose to confront, avoid, or tolerate.

Toleration is really a form of avoiding the issue. It doesn't show true care.

Avoidance is really for your benefit. It keeps you from getting out of your comfort zone.

Confronting sounds harsh, but I'm talking about an encouraging, comforting telling of truth in the appropriate time, place, and manner. The challenge is knowing the right time. If you fail to communicate the truth in a timely fashion it may indeed be too late for that person to heal.

By being too nice and doing things that you perceive other people want you to do leaves you in a scenario that isn't displaying truth or God's love. Tolerating their sin can usually lead to deeper despair or struggles.

What I love about the surgeon is that he communicated his call through action, which is what I am striving to do.

Where do you need to be the surgeon for Christ?

_____

_____

_____

However my parents, relatives and friends have all given gentle warnings and signs to help guide my path. I didn't always listen, so sometimes a more stern approach really could be warranted.

Do you remember someone who conveyed truth even though you didn't want to hear it? Did they display it in action?

_____

_____

_____

_____

How did they do it?

_____

_____

_____

_____

Is there someone in your life that God may be prompting you to share 'Revival care' with to bring truth to them?

_____

_____

_____

_____

_____

What Bible verses support that care and focus for them? (this is your time to do some searches and find something that God is speaking to you through) Check out your Bible or search Biblegateway.org

_____

_____

_____

_____

_____

What true care do you need to show to others?

_____

_____

_____

_____

_____

Refreshment is the essence of courage. Taking on a task or a goal and working with all your energy towards success is captivating, intriguing and motivating. It super charges forces around you and hones your motivation. However anytime you start something there is an inherent risk associated with it that the outcomes may not be in line with your desire.

Life is risk, and it gets riskier if we try to do it on our own.

A colleague and friend at work, Jack, also likes to say, and "encouraging courage" as something we are striving to do with some of our initiatives on the job. In the trainings we have coordinated together we have striven to live and communicate that courage in everything we have done. "To encourage courage" is a simple catchy phrase that captivates bravery in the face of trials, overcoming adversity as an underdog, uplifting others to achieve the greatness that God has outlined for them.

I think of the life of Biblical David when he faced the giant. In 1 Samuel 17:43-46, David's words show the depth of strength and confirm where his reliance was.

"David said to the Philistine (Goliath), 'You come against me with sword and spear and javelin, but I come against you in the name of the Lord Almighty, the God of the armies of Israel, who you have defied. This day the Lord will deliver you into my hands."

Prior to taking this risk he spoke to Saul about whether he should enter into battle. Saul tried to talk David out of it, but after Saul had tested David's resolve and sheer and utter confidence in the Lord, he tried to put his armor on David. But David refused and did as he felt led by God to do.

Imagine the nervousness that the entire group of people must have felt. If David was your son or your sibling, would you have let him go into battle against a blood thirsty, professional giant of a warrior?

What 'Goliath' in your life is coming out and taunting you daily? What do you need to let go of and put your trust in Jesus about?

_____

_____

_____

_____

My friend, Jack, also modified a quote that he modified from another famous one that I love. "Anything worth doing, is worth doing poorly."

As he puts, it you've probably heard the saying that "Anything worth doing, is worth doing well." His rational to modify that quote is with the highlight and the focus that sometimes we may not risk doing something because we may not be able to do it well.

I agree there is definitely a time for skill building and

precision. But in developing your baseline and establishing a springboard to excel from, it's more important to do something even if you do it poorly or completely fail.

Some may argue that it's about the form, the precision, etc. But think of a child learning to walk. At first they stand up, collapse, fall, and roll so many times. If anyone has ever counted it wouldn't surprise me to see them fall over 1000 times before they are able to function. If it did take 1000 times, the first 1 means that child is 999 times closer to success.

This is a hard reminder for us as we age and are more conscientious about what we do.

Through the journey to better health for myself, I have risked failing and looking uncoordinated attending classes I would have never normally attended before at the club. I don't even know what the names mean, but I went optimistically and always told myself that'd I'd try it 21 days to get the cobwebs out and better adapt to the class.

Amazingly, the process was always the same. First excitement, then reality sets in, hard work and adaptation. These phases of adaptation are similar to when you come into a new work environment or a new culture where you are seeking out how to interact and connect with the individuals.

At first excitement for the new task and skill. It's a new time, with new people, and new aches and pains. After the first two or three times there is a realization that it is much tougher than it looks and that my coordination and form is at the level of a beginner.

When I watch the instructor doing the exercise holding three to five times the weight as me, speaking and coaching the crowd effortlessly, yet barely breaking a sweat, I hesitate to ask them how long they have been doing this. One instructor and trainer mentioned that she has been leading the class. For over thirteen years. If my math is right that is 13x50= at least 650 times if she only did one class per week. The reality is that some weeks she said she might lead three classes per day amidst the other nine classes she is running in a week.

Then comes the hard work and I've found that if I desire to do it, I usually can master it after seven to ten class sessions. A good instructor usually brings in new variations so it never seems like the same routine. They keep mixing it up.

For me it takes about one to three months typically I can hang with the best of them. That is when I am closer to the adaptation and assimilation phase. I know the moves, the lingo, and when the variation comes in I am more ready to adapt. The first time I ever went to one of these classes was in college as I was always what seemed like two steps behind in the routine. So I gave it up for fifteen years and relegated myself to running and bicycling as I felt too vulnerable and told myself that coordinated moves such as these were not something I could do.

As you can see, my negative self-talk channeled me into a state of being that left me talking myself out of even trying. Don't let this type of negativity keep you from trying new things. If you don't try, you'll never improve. Yes even now there are some moves that the instructor does and I just laugh internally as I know I am the only one in the room who seems out of synchronization.

Think of the benefits of trying and falling. For that child it's one step closer to success and necessary in the process of growth. So I know that if doing the classes or exercises are worthwhile, I am willing to fail and be the slower or out-of-sync person in the class, with the knowledge that I am one step closer to success.

Matthew 11:25-30 is awesome:

"At that time Jesus said, "I praise you, Father, Lord of heaven and earth, because you have hidden these things from the wise and learned, and revealed them to little children. 26 Yes, Father, for this is what you were pleased to do.

²⁷ "All things have been committed to me by my Father. No one knows the Son except the Father, and no one knows the Father except the Son and those to whom the Son chooses to reveal him.

²⁸ "Come to me, all you who are weary and burdened, and I will give you rest. ²⁹ Take my yoke upon you and learn from me, for I am gentle and humble in heart, and you will find rest for your souls. ³⁰ For my yoke is easy and my burden is light."

Is the yoke Christ has given you easy?

_____

_____

_____

_____

If not, how are you getting in the way of Christ?

_____

_____

_____

_____

From Roman's 7:4-25

"So, my brothers and sisters, you also died to the law through the body of Christ, that you might belong to another, to him who was raised from the dead, in order that we might bear fruit for God. For when we were in the realm of the flesh, the sinful passions aroused by the law were at work in us, so that we bore fruit for death. But now, by dying to what once bound us, we have been released from the law so that we serve in the new way of the Spirit, and not in the old way of the written code.

What shall we say, then? Is the law sinful? Certainly not! Nevertheless, I would not have known what sin was had it not been for the law. For I would not have known what coveting really was if the law had not said, "You shall not covet." But sin, seizing the opportunity afforded by the commandment, produced in me every kind of coveting. For apart from the law, sin was dead. Once I was alive apart from the law; but when the commandment came, sin sprang to life and I died. I found that the very commandment that was intended to bring life actually brought death. For sin, seizing the opportunity afforded by the commandment, deceived me, and through the commandment put me to death. So then, the law is holy, and the commandment is holy, righteous and good.

Did that which is good, then, become death to me? By no means! Nevertheless, in order that sin might be recognized as sin, it used what is good to bring about my death, so that through the commandment sin might become utterly sinful.

We know that the law is spiritual; but I am unspiritual, sold as a slave to sin. I do not understand what I do. For what I want to do I do not do, but what I hate I do. And if I do what I do not want to do, I agree that the law is good. As it is, it is no longer I myself who do it, but it is sin living in me. For I know that good itself does not dwell in me, that is, in my sinful nature. For I have the desire to do what is good, but I cannot carry it out. For I do not do the good I want to do, but the evil I do not want to do—this I keep on doing. Now if I do what I do not want to do, it is no longer I who do it, but it is sin living in me that does it.

So I find this law at work: Although I want to do good, evil is right there with me. For in my inner being I delight in God's law; but I see another law at work in me, waging war against the law of my mind and making me a prisoner of the law of sin at work within me. What a wretched man I am! Who will rescue me from this body that is subject to death? Thanks be to God, who delivers me through Jesus Christ our Lord!

So then, I myself in my mind am a slave to God's law, but in my sinful nature a slave to the law of sin. "

Wow! Isn't that enough said.

Knowing that we are bound in our nature by sin, and Christ is the only answer is so freeing. It allows us to move forward with greater and deeper faith. Please don't get down on yourself if you do something wrong, or poorly, just move on to Christ and ask for His forgiveness.

Please don't hold grudges against others. Move on with Christ and forgive them as He has forgiven you. We should get busy doing the Lord's work as we are called to do.

But be judicious and steadfast in what you are busy doing. Do what is important to achieving what He is guiding you to discover.

What stands out in those verses that you need to apply to your life right now?

_____

_____

_____

Psalm 27 also is a capstone verse that could encourage your growth and strength.

The LORD is my light and my salvation—
whom shall I fear?
The LORD is the stronghold of my life—
of whom shall I be afraid?

When the wicked advance against me
to devour me,
it is my enemies and my foes
who will stumble and fall.
Though an army besiege me,
my heart will not fear;
though war break out against me,
even then I will be confident.

One thing I ask from the LORD,
this only do I seek:
that I may dwell in the house of the LORD
all the days of my life,
to gaze on the beauty of the LORD

and to seek him in his temple.
For in the day of trouble
he will keep me safe in his dwelling;
he will hide me in the shelter of his sacred tent
and set me high upon a rock.

Then my head will be exalted
above the enemies who surround me;
at his sacred tent I will sacrifice with shouts of joy;
I will sing and make music to the LORD.

Hear my voice when I call, LORD;
be merciful to me and answer me.
My heart says of you, "Seek his face!"
Your face, LORD, I will seek.
Do not hide your face from me,
do not turn your servant away in anger;
you have been my helper.
Do not reject me or forsake me,
God my Savior.
Though my father and mother forsake me,
the LORD will receive me.
Teach me your way, LORD;
lead me in a straight path
because of my oppressors.
Do not turn me over to the desire of my foes,
for false witnesses rise up against me,
spouting malicious accusations.

I remain confident of this:
I will see the goodness of the LORD
in the land of the living.
Wait for the LORD;
be strong and take heart
and wait for the LORD.

What do you need to apply from this verse?

Remember the only thing things that we know go into Heaven are God, His Word and the Saved. Live for Him, His Word and praise Him for saving you.

Many blessings to you.

D. Duane Engler

Appendix

Some thoughts:

What thoughts do you meditate on to get you groovin', to get you movin', to get you in gear to achieve?

_____

_____

_____

_____

_____

_____

Positive Revival Diet™ thoughts and verse to keep motivation alive:

> *"Therefore do not worry about tomorrow, for tomorrow will worry about itself. Each day has enough trouble of its own."*
> Matthew 6:34

> *"I can do all this through him who gives me strength."*
> Philippians 4:13

> *"Those who hope in the LORD will renew their strength. They will soar on wings like eagles; they will run and not grow weary, they will walk and not be faint."*
> Isaiah 40:31

> *"Therefore I tell you, do not worry about your life, what you will eat or drink; or about your body, what you will wear. Is not life more than food, and the body more than clothes? Look at the birds of the air; they do not sow or reap or store away in barns, and yet your heavenly Father feeds them. Are you not much more valuable than*

they? Can any one of you by worrying add a single hour to your life?"

Matthew 6:25-27

"But make up your mind not to worry beforehand how you will defend yourselves."

Luke 21:14

"Cast your cares on the LORD and he will sustain you; he will never let the righteous be shaken."

Psalm 55:22

"For the Spirit God gave us does not make us timid, but gives us power, love and self-discipline."

2 Timothy 1:7

"I keep my eyes always on the LORD. With him at my right hand, I will not be shaken.".

Psalm 16:8

"Truly he is my rock and my salvation; he is my fortress, I will not be shaken."

Psalm 62:6

"Keep me as the apple of your eye; hide me in the shadow of your wings"

Psalm 17:8

"He will cover you with his feathers, and under his wings you will find refuge; his faithfulness will be your shield and rampart."

Psalm 91:4

"So do not fear, for I am with you; do not be dismayed, for I am your God. I will strengthen you and help you; I will uphold you with my righteous right hand."

    Isaiah 41:10

"For I know the plans I have for you," declares the LORD, "plans to prosper you and not to harm you, plans to give you hope and a future."

    Jeremiah 29:11

"And we know that in all things God works for the good of those who love him, who have been called according to his purpose."

    Romans 8:28

"The LORD is my strength and my shield; my heart trusts in him, and he helps me.

    Psalm 28:7

"I lift up my eyes to the mountains— where does my help come from? My help comes from the LORD, the Maker of heaven and earth."

    Psalm 121:1-2

    *(I love mountains so this one really inspires me)

"They will have no fear of bad news; their hearts are steadfast, trusting in the LORD.

    Psalm 112:7

"Trust in the LORD with all your heart and lean not on your own understanding"

    Proverbs 3:5-6

"There you saw how the LORD your God carried you, as a father carries his son, all the way you went until you reached this place.
Deuteronomy 1:31

"Do not be anxious about anything, but in every situation, by prayer and petition, with thanksgiving, present your requests to God. And the peace of God, which transcends all understanding, will guard your hearts and your minds in Christ Jesus."
Philippians4:6-7

"I have fought the good fight, I have finished the race, I have kept the faith."
2   Timothy 4:7

"Therefore, since we are surrounded by such a great cloud of witnesses, let us throw off everything that hinders and the sin that so easily entangles. And let us run with perseverance the race marked out for us, fixing our eyes on Jesus, the pioneer and perfecter of faith. For the joy set before him he endured the cross, scorning its shame, and sat down at the right hand of the throne of God."
Hebrews 12:1-2

"God is our refuge and strength, an ever-present help in trouble."
Psalm 46:1

"Do not let your hearts be troubled. You believe in God; believe also in me."
John 14:1

"Come to me, all you who are weary and burdened, and I will give you rest. Take my yoke upon you and learn from me, for I am gentle and humble in heart, and you will find rest for your souls. For my yoke is easy and my burden is light."
Matthew 11:28-30

"When I am afraid, I put my trust in you."
Psalm 56:3

"Be strong and courageous. Do not be afraid or terrified because of them, for the LORD your God goes with you; he will never leave you nor forsake you."
Deuteronomy 31:6

"Am I now trying to win the approval of human beings, or of God? Or am I trying to please people? If I were still trying to please people, I would not be a servant of Christ."
Galatians 1:10

"What, then, shall we say in response to these things? If God is for us, who can be against us?"
Romans 8:31

"Know also that wisdom is like honey for you: If you find it, there is a future hope for you, and your hope will not be cut off."
Proverbs 24:14

"I prayed to the LORD, and he answered me. He freed me from all my fears. Those who look to him for help will be radiant with joy; no shadow of shame will darken their faces. In my desperation I prayed, and the LORD listened; he saved me from all my troubles. For the angel of the LORD is a guard; he surrounds and defends all who fear him."
Psalm 34:4-7

"Give all your worries and cares to God, for he cares about you. Stay alert! Watch out for your great enemy, the devil. He prowls around like a roaring lion, looking for someone to devour. Stand

firm against him, and be strong in your faith. Remember that your Christian brothers and sisters all over the world are going through the same kind of suffering you are. In his kindness God called you to share in his eternal glory by means of Christ Jesus. So after you have suffered a little while, he will restore, support, and strengthen you, and he will place you on a firm foundation."

1 Peter 5:7-10

"As for God, his way is perfect: The LORD's word is flawless; he shields all who take refuge in him."

2   Samuel 22:31

"Come to me, all you who are weary and burdened, and I will give you rest. Take my yoke upon you and learn from me, for I am gentle and humble in heart, and you will find rest for your souls. For my yoke is easy and my burden is light."

Matthew 11:28-30

"The LORD is my strength and my defense; he has become my salvation. He is my God, and I will praise him, my father's God, and I will exalt him."

Exodus 15:2

"We have this hope as an anchor for the soul, firm and secure."

Hebrews 6:19

"The mind governed by the flesh is death, but the mind governed by the Spirit is life and peace."

Romans 8:6

"Peace I leave with you; my peace I give you. I do not give to you as the world gives. Do not let your hearts be troubled and do not be afraid."

John 14:27

"May the God who gives endurance and encouragement give you the same attitude of mind toward each other that Christ Jesus had, so that with one mind and one voice you may glorify the God and Father of our Lord Jesus Christ."

Romans 15:5-6

"You were taught, with regard to your former way of life, to put off your old self, which is being corrupted by its deceitful desires; to be made new in the attitude of your minds; and to put on the new self, created to be like God in true righteousness and holiness."

Romans 4:22-24

"My flesh and my heart may fail, but God is the strength of my heart and my portion forever."

Psalm 73:26

"Because of the LORD's great love we are not consumed, for his compassions never fail. They are new every morning; great is your faithfulness."

Lamentations 3:22-23

"For the word of God is alive and active. Sharper than any double-edged sword, it penetrates even to dividing soul and spirit, joints and marrow; it judges the thoughts and attitudes of the heart."

Hebrews 4:12

"What, then, shall we say in response to these things? If God is for us, who can be against us?"

Romans 8:31

"As for God, his way is perfect: The LORD's word is flawless; he shields all who take refuge in him."

Psalm 18:30

"Are God's consolations not enough for you, words spoken gently to you?"

Job 15:11

"The righteous cry out, and the LORD hears them; he delivers them from all their troubles. The LORD is close to the brokenhearted and saves those who are crushed in spirit. The righteous person may have many troubles, but the LORD delivers him from them all."

Psalm 34:17-19

"Guide me in your truth and teach me, for you are God my Savior, and my hope is in you all day long."

Psalm 25:5

"They will be like a tree planted by the water that sends out its roots by the stream. It does not fear when heat comes; its leaves are always green. It has no worries in a year of drought and never fails to bear fruit."

Jeremiah 17:8

"For the word of the LORD is right and true; he is faithful in all he does. The LORD loves righteousness and justice; the earth is full of his unfailing love."

Psalm 33:4-5

Other personal mantras and quotes I use to keep going:

"I can do this"

"The lonely work will get me through"

"After I start I will adapt and learn"

"I need to achieve success one day, one hour, one minute, one second at a time"

"Don't think too much about it, just get 'er going"

"When I'm done I'm going to celebrate by enjoying a hot tub time"

"I will only strive to make it the next minute"

"I'm going to count laps like years of history backwards, considering each century and what I know about what happened in the world during those years in the areas of cultural, global, innovations and events"

"Pain is temporary and will make you stronger"

James 1 (need I say more)

"Honoring God is my goal"

"The healthier food tastes better. Why settle for junk? Wait for the best nutrient rich foods"

"I have self control"

"I will feel better"

"I will limit my dead foods"

"God will revive and refresh my soul"

"I will turn away from worldly, fleeting temporary, things and focus on eternity"

"I will sleep better knowing I've done my best"

"I am helping people"

"This will make me wiser and stronger"

"I prefer the healthier choice versus the counterfeit choice"

"Quitting is forever, pain is temporary – keep going"

Reality = A + B + C + D + E

Please write down your current reality (use extra paper if you'd like too): *these equations are also listed on convenient pages in the back of the book you can print off)

_____

=

_____

+

_____

+

_____

+

_____

Now write the new life that you are striving for has a desired outcome and the simple equation is to substitute the items that make your current reality by the outcomes that will get you to your desired Life.

Desired Life = G + O + D

_____

=

_____

+

_____

+

_____

Item
Original Ingredients   **Christian Revival**
                                  Diet™ Substitutions

_____

_____

_____

_____

_____

_____

_____

_____

_____

_____

_____

_____

_____

_____

_____

_____

Similar size
Calories =   Calories =
Cost =   Cost =
Questionable nutritional content Nutrient Packed
                                  Christian   Revival
                                  Food™

I'd love to hear from you with any experimental Christian
Revival Food™ that you have discovered. Send me an email:
engler21@gmail.com

Psalm 23

The LORD *is my shepherd, I lack nothing.*
2 He makes me lie down in green pastures,
he leads me beside quiet waters,
3 he refreshes my soul.
He guides me along the right paths
for his name's sake.
4 Even though I walk
through the darkest valley,
I will fear no evil,
for you are with me;
your rod and your staff,
they comfort me.

5 You prepare a table before me
in the presence of my enemies.
You anoint my head with oil;
my cup overflows.
6 Surely your goodness and love will follow me
all the days of my life,
and I will dwell in the house of the LORD
forever.

ABOUT THE AUTHOR

D. Duane Engler is a son, husband, father, and a friend. He loves the Lord and seeks to work to Him in all he does, although often falling short.

He has led and been involved in many ministry activities: Bible Study Fellowship, Men's 1-1 Discipleship, fellowship with family and friends in God's nature.

As a professional educator, coach and speaker D. Duane aims to help others live out Proverbs 4:26 as they consider the paths of their feet.

D. Duane resides in Edina, Minnesota, where he is working on his next book.

May you be a blessing!

James 1: 2-8

*"Consider it pure joy, my brothers and sisters, whenever you face trials of many kinds, ³ because you know that the testing of your faith produces perseverance. ⁴ Let perseverance finish its work so that you may be mature and complete, not lacking anything. ⁵ If any of you lacks wisdom, you should ask God, who gives generously to all without finding fault, and it will be given to you. ⁶ **But when you ask, you must believe and not doubt**, because the one who doubts is like a wave of the sea, blown and tossed by the wind. ⁷*
That person should not expect to receive anything from the Lord. ⁸ Such a person is double-minded and unstable in all they do."

www.ingramcontent.com/pod-product-compliance
Lightning Source LLC
Chambersburg PA
CBHW060454290526
45791CB00001B/117